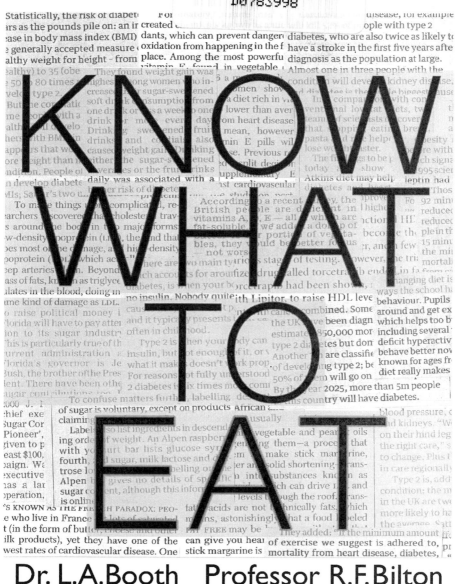

KNOW WHAT TO EAT

Dr. L.A.Booth   Professor R.F. Bilton

Published by Supercritical,
25 Victoria Road,
Formby,
Merseyside
L37 7AQ

First edition 2013

A CIP catalogue record for this title is available from the British
Library.

ISBN 978-0-9567366-1-1

Printed and bound in Great Britain by Azimuth Print Ltd

We wish to thank our families for their patience, support and input. Rod wishes to thank his sons for their substantial input, particularly in completing the final copy. Dr Mark Bilton and Joseph Bilton (Msc) helped with the editing and formatting of the final text, and thanks to Joseph for the cover design. Finally, our particular thanks go to Dr Peter Barnes for his invaluable experience in food related scientific publishing, and also his enthusiastic support and encouragement.

CONTENTS

Preface

Knowledge is the key to understanding how the human body works, and how to minimise the risk of diseases common in the industrial world such as obesity, diabetes, cancer and heart disease. Although health is largely determined by lifestyle, eating healthy foods is not as easy as it sounds. The complexity of choice is bewildering. Misleading information and aggressive but subtle marketing has led to confusion in the minds of the public.

As academic biochemists we have extensively researched the scientific literature and worked in the laboratory to better understand the workings of living cells and the human body. It is the immense gulf between the scientific understanding of health issues and the public perception that has moved us to write this book. For example, the following statements are still seen in the popular press: 'butter is bad, margarine is good', 'saturated fat is bad', 'blood cholesterol must be lowered' and 'every male over 50 years of age in the UK should be taking statins'. In each case there is no reputable science to support these statements. The stark truth is that the food and pharmaceutical industries would rather you remained reliant upon their products for life instead of making basic lifestyle changes to achieve good health. Too much power lies in the hands of these extremely profitable industries.

We provide information on the types of foods that optimise good health and an ideal body mass, and those that should be avoided. Controversies concerning diet and health are examined in detail with reference to the current obesity and diabetes epidemics, and the conflicting interests of the food and drug industries and the consumer. Facts from recent leading-edge research and past undervalued discoveries explain the crises in modern nutrition.

1 Historical links between diet and disease

Introduction

The idea that nutrition is an important factor in the development of many chronic diseases is not new. Some Roman physicians were convinced that people who regularly ate cabbage were less likely to develop certain forms of cancer. In China towards the end of the first millennium, it was recognised that poor nutrition was a cause of oesophageal cancer. Ancient Hindu texts identified that the symptoms of diabetes were most commonly seen in the upper classes of society, i.e. those on a sugar-rich diet. Coronary heart disease (CHD), another disease of affluence which is common today, has been detected in mummies from Egypt and Peru, as evidenced by hardening of the arteries (calcified deposits) in the blood vessels of the heart observed in mummified remains. In contrast to popular belief, the infamous Rameses the Second suffered from advanced arteriosclerosis in his old age and probably died of a heart attack, rather than 'drowning', the explanation of his death offered in the Bible.

Over the past 300 years, members of the medical profession in the UK have observed the connections between diet, obesity, diabetes, cancer and several chronic diseases. Wiseman in 1676 suggested that the consumption of salt, 'sharp' and 'gross' meats might cause cancer, and in 1811 Howard proposed that constipation was a possible cause of bowel cancer. In 1815 Lambe, a member of the Royal College of Physicians in London, warned that overconsumption of food in general and meat in particular was a cause of cancer and other chronic diseases [1], and Bennett in 1849 associated overeating and obesity with increased cancer risk.

During the 1860s, a clinically obese Victorian named William Banting gained fame and notoriety in the UK for achieving rapid weight loss. He took dietary advice from William Harvey, a physician, who had previously proposed a link between diabetes, obesity and dietary carbohydrate, and had embarked on a low carbohydrate diet. He lost 46lb in the first year and his joint problems, hearing and sight greatly improved. His pamphlet extolling the virtues of this pre-Atkins Diet[1] sold 50,000 copies amongst the diet-conscious Victorians. The medical profession of his day was antagonistic, questioning his methods and even pronounced him dead before his time, citing his 'unhealthy' diet as the cause [2]. The contemporary medical establishment is similarly critical of the efficacy of the Atkins-type diets.

By the early part of the twentieth century, the view that diet can cause chronic disease was common amongst physicians. In 1907 Shaw came up with a very prudent low-risk diet with increased vegetable intake and reductions in animal food products, alcohol, tea and tobacco. This prescient advice is just as relevant today. In 1908, Williams stressed the dangers of gluttony and lack of exercise in the development of chronic diseases, yet articles in the media present these ideas as something new.

The emerging consensus

In 1937 a review of the available literature of diet and cancer by a founder member of the American Cancer Society, Dr Frederic Hoffman, concluded that excessive eating, if not a primary cause,

---

[1] Banting may have been the inspiration for several subsequent low carbohydrate diets for weight loss, with *Eat Fat and Grow Slim* by Dr Richard Mackarness in 1958 and the Atkins Diet gaining prominence in the 1980s.

is a leading factor in the development of cancer. Hoffman identified fatty, sugary foods [3], white bread and meat as important potential risk factors.

In the UK during the Second World War and the years that followed, a significant decrease in the occurrence of Type 2 diabetes was observed. This may have been a consequence of the scarcity of sugar during those difficult times in Europe. Those in the UK old enough to remember the period will recall the ration books and lack of sugar and sweets until the early 1950s.

When Ancel Keys visited Crete in the 1950s to research the Mediterranean diet, cancer and heart disease, he was astounded to find that there were no specialist hospital facilities for those ailments. Furthermore, most of the population obtained a minimum of 40% of their daily calories from fat [4]. Heart disease and cancer were virtually unknown on the island at that time. What Keys did discover was that the dietary fat was largely unrefined olive oil, carbohydrate intake was complex in association with fibre in wholemeal bread, and large amounts of fruit and vegetables were consumed, together with moderate amounts of fish and white meat. Red meat was eaten infrequently and wine consumption was moderate. This combination can hardly be improved on today and is the basis for the proven efficacy of a Mediterranean style diet. Keys went on to propose that dietary saturated fat was the principal cause of obesity and heart disease.

The great nutritionist Professor John Yudkin, who initiated the study of nutrition at university level in the UK, had already proposed in 1957 that dietary sugar was the major risk factor in heart disease, diabetes and obesity. When his book *Pure, White and Deadly* was published in 1972, there was an outcry from the powerful food industry lobby, and their associated academics, Keys included, and an attempt to discredit his important research. Yudkin's work has since been vindicated in worldwide studies, but this has done nothing to curb the excesses of the sugar industry, as discussed in Chapter 3.

In the second half of the 20th century, significant changes took place. Theories concerning the dietary origins of cancer were largely discounted. Instead, the theories of random genetic error and exposure to viruses or specific cancer-causing chemicals gained in popularity. Research in the field of cancer and chronic disease underwent a major shift towards investigations into the cellular and molecular origins of cancer. Surgery, chemotherapy and radiotherapy became the accepted treatments for cancer.

In the developed world, life expectancy greatly increased. Death rates from infectious diseases fell sharply as a result of improved medical treatment and antibiotic therapy. People were now living much longer and as a consequence had a greater exposure to environmental pollution, unhealthy diets and the effects of inactivity. This situation rekindled interest in the nutritional causes of cancer.

In 1969, Burkitt presented his seminal hypothesis on the role of low fibre 'Western diets' in increasing the incidence of colon cancer. Meanwhile, in the United States, Richard Nixon declared that defeating cancer was a national goal, equivalent in importance to putting a man on the moon.

In 1977, a scientific review suggested that diet accounted for 40% of all male cancers and 60% of all female cancers [5]. This study also suggested that one of the key causes of these cancers was overeating. Four years later, further studies suggested that dietary modification might reduce cancer deaths in the US by as much as an average of 35% [6]. The diet that these scientists refer to is high in fat and refined carbohydrates whilst low in fibre and essential vitamins and minerals. This gives new hope to people intent on reducing their risk of cancer and chronic disease and to governments of countries whose expenditure on cancer and chronic disease treatment is becoming an additional financial burden to already over-stretched health services.

In March 2003, the World Health Organisation (WHO) produced a report on diet, nutrition and prevention of the chronic diseases cancer, CHD and diabetes. The most significant recommendation in the discussion document (published on the internet), and tellingly missing from the final document, was the recommendation that no more than 10% of daily calories should be derived from added sugar. The original unabridged report caused political turmoil and evoked fury among the sugar-producing nations and sections of the food industry. This report reviewed worldwide research indicating that the major factors in the incidence of diseases such as heart disease, diabetes, obesity and cancer in the developed world are the consumption of too much sugar-rich food and lack of physical exercise.

Understanding the relationship between diet and disease is not simple. The complexity arises because there are a large number of diseases and a wide variety of diets. This complexity may be unravelled by studying the relationship between disease incidence and specific diets. Two well-known examples of this are the low levels of heart disease and colon cancer in traditional Eskimos (Inuit), and colorectal cancer in American Seventh Day Adventists, who eat a mainly vegetarian diet. In addition, first generation Japanese immigrants to Hawaii retaining their dietary and cultural habits maintained a low incidence of cancer and heart disease; subsequent generations adopting the modern

5

American lifestyle acquired the typical American higher disease rates for obesity, diabetes, heart disease and cancer.

An extra level of complexity is added by the different approaches taken by scientists in their studies of diet and disease. Nevertheless, scientific study into the relationship between diet and disease has made significant headway, and a large volume of scientific information and recommendation exists. Paramount in diet and disease research has been the finding that diets high in fruit and vegetables, and their associated antioxidants and bioactive micronutrients, are associated with a reduced risk of the development of most cancers, CHD and obesity [5, 6]. This is explained in detail later in Chapter 7.

Development of the human diet

All air-breathing creatures have a highly efficient, oxygen-based system of respiration. However, oxygen can be toxic and forms damaging free radicals, which are normally destroyed by protective enzymes.[2] In the distant past, the plant kingdom had to develop a sophisticated antioxidant defence system against atmospheric oxygen toxicity. Herbivorous and omnivorous animals, including humans, have effectively hijacked these systems for their own survival. Plants are a rich source of both oil- and water-soluble antioxidant pigments and vitamins, which play a crucial role in both metabolic processes and cellular protective mechanisms. These dietary elements may help to reduce the incidence of cell mutation, cancer and heart disease. In recent years, studies have confirmed that diets rich in fruit,

---

[2] The Appendix outlines how free radicals are formed, how they can damage cells, and how the body defends itself against these highly reactive molecules.

vegetable and whole grains provide a high level of these protective dietary components [5, 6].

Modern man, *Homo sapiens,* appeared as a distinct species some 100,000 years ago. Racial groups may have changed gradually over the years but the essential human genome was complete all those thousands of years ago. Most important is the fact that the human body had already evolved to digest and metabolise food in exactly the same way we do today. However, there is a great difference between what our ancestors ate and our current diet. Our immediate pre-sapiens ancestor *Homo erectus* was more closely related to our common ape-like forebears in having teeth designed to chew vegetable matter. Fossil skeleton remains also indicate the presence of a very large stomach and gut necessary for the digestion of plant material. Modern anthropologists suggest that the evolution to *Homo sapiens* involved the transition from a herbivorous to a carnivorous diet, as modern man's teeth are more characteristic of a carnivore; the much smaller stomach and gut required for the energy-dense carnivore diet means that more energy could be diverted to the development of the brain.

This may be the reason for the displacement of Neanderthal man from Northern Europe in the ice ages. Although the Neanderthal had a massive skeleton that could support the large weight of fat needed to survive the Arctic winters, *Homo sapiens* with a much slighter frame was probably better able to withstand the cold because of the ability to sew animal skins into clothing. Some anthropologists [7] have argued that our early ancestors lived primarily on the aquatic margins by the sea and along rivers and lakes. This would not only allow travel by boat away from predators in the dense forests, but gave them easy access to an abundant food source of fish and shellfish.

7

Fish diets are rich in the long chain omega-3 fats which are crucial in the development of a large brain. By comparison, animals in the continental savannahs and forests have relatively low levels of omega-3 fats in their diets and much smaller brain mass/body ratios than humans. Early *Homo sapiens* survived by fishing, hunting and gathering fruits and vegetables. The fact that the land was untamed by agriculture meant that finding food often required energetic pursuit of game, often over many miles with extensive searches for fruits and vegetables. The life of these early hunter gatherers was of necessity highly active and highly dependent on the seasonal changes in food availability. In colder climes, winter presented more problems with dramatic decreases in the abundance of food so that Palaeolithic man periodically experienced partial and total starvation. Feeding was sporadic with no guarantee of food in the immediate future; the human body, as a consequence, became highly efficient at extracting and storing energy and nutrients from food.

It has been proposed by Linus Pauling that our ancestors were decimated in the ice ages not by the cold, but because of the lack of vitamin C. Vitamin C deficiency was also prevalent among sailors, causing scurvy, often resulting in internal haemorrhaging from leaking blood vessels. Captain Cook found that limes prevented this condition and originated the nickname of 'limies'. The elderly often do not absorb sufficient dietary vitamin C to maintain arterial integrity and have an increased risk of cardiovascular diseases (CVD). Vitamin C deficiency may also contribute to the epidemic rise of heart disease in inactive populations on junk food diets.

An analysis of the types of food eaten by our ancestors shows a predominance of natural food rich in protein, fat and micronutrients and no refined carbohydrates or excessive

8

consumption of salt. Fat was extremely important as an energy source, much more so than it is today, and was highly prized by our active ancestors. The little sugar consumed in the Palaeolithic diet was present in ripe fruit, tubers and honey. Compared with the quantity of sugar consumed today in the developed world, the amount was miniscule.

The discovery of fire enabled our ancestors to cook food, making meat softer and roots and tubers more digestible. Smoking of meat and fish allowed the storage of protein-rich food. Approximately 10,000 years ago, simple agriculture began to develop. Cultivation and storage of cereals, roots, tubers and pulses enabled people to congregate in towns and villages. Grains were processed, then dried and stored or used for making bread and other foods. Man was becoming less nomadic and storage of food meant a better chance of survival in the winter season. In effect, what humans were now doing was storing their food in shelters over the winter instead of as fat around their waists. Hunting was less of a necessity, but would have complemented the diet of these early farmers. The cultivation of grains meant a significant change in man's diet, with considerably more carbohydrates being consumed. It is interesting to speculate as to whether the adoption of cereals as a major food source at this time was the beginning of the problems associated with obesity and cereal allergies. Around the same time, the domestication of animals began, many of which were bred for food. In addition, people living in villages close to water would have eaten relatively large amounts of fresh fish. Very recently fish eating has declined, particularly in the US and the UK.

Our present way of living has only become typical within the past two generations. Diets consumed in modern industrialised countries today have evolved considerably from those of our early Stone Age ancestors. It was the industrial revolution that completely altered our diet, along with the shift of populations from the country to towns and the limited access of town dwellers to fruits, vegetables and other fresh foods.

Foods such as highly refined white sugar and white flour, which used to be common only in the diets of the wealthy, became mass produced and were readily accessible. Many of these foods were highly refined and processed to yield large scale production of a uniform product, which led to food containing less fibre, vitamins and minerals, in a less nutritional product. Refined cane sugar was used in cakes, biscuits, confectionery, chocolate, jams and soft drinks: foods once only consumed by the rich, with the resultant obesity, diabetes and gout. Modern cheap processed foods have the potential to increase these ailments in most sections of society, especially since we are probably even less active than our wealthy forebears. Changes in lifestyle and diet, especially the increased consumption of processed junk foods, have resulted in the extremely unhealthy modern society we have today: we are Stone Age hunter gatherers in a world vastly different to that for which our constitution evolved.

The only remaining examples of Stone Age type cultures today are the traditional Inuit who have a very low incidence of heart disease and cancer on their fish-rich diets, but this is fast changing with the adoption of cola and ice cream as the junk food culture spreads north. Stone Age cultures of the inaccessible forests of New Guinea may have healthy mixed diets, but their study has proved too hazardous.

Many diet-related diseases in developed countries are a direct consequence of our very efficient 100,000 year old metabolic processes being overwhelmed by an excess of readily available calories from junk food diets. However, it must be stressed that processed food is not the only source of the problem. Overconsumption of healthy foods with excess calories will also lead to the same metabolic disturbances. The food eaten during our lifetime is directly linked to our long-term health, in terms of both the quality and quantity consumed. Several nutritional studies with creatures ranging from fruit flies to rats have clearly demonstrated that total calorie consumption is related to lifespan. Without exception, the restriction of specific food types and therefore the restriction of specific calorie intake gave substantial increases in longevity.

2   Human metabolism

Before informed decisions can be made about which foods will be good or bad for our health, some background knowledge is needed on how our bodies digest and metabolise (break down) the food we eat.

The human body has evolved an exquisite mechanism for withstanding partial and prolonged starvation. How this ability impacts on the diet-related health concerns of modern society will be outlined. How the crucial hormone insulin is involved in the major diseases of modern society, coronary heart disease, diabetes, cancer and obesity, is also explained.

Metabolism: the basics

The food we eat is broken down by the digestive system and then absorbed by the body. Once absorbed from the gut into the blood, the digested food is metabolised first by the liver and then by the other organs. Metabolism includes all the processes that occur in the body which change and use the products of digestion. Food is digested into a form that can be used by our bodies for energy and growth; this is the purpose of metabolism. All of the foods we eat, except insoluble fibre, are metabolised and all have different functions within the body. Metabolism and metabolic rates (the rates at which we use the food we eat) vary from person to person. This explains why different people on the same diet can vary considerably in body mass and why some diets are unsuitable for some people.

Here the focus is on the basic features of human metabolism. Current research on diet and metabolism using sophisticated, state of the art techniques has reached an exciting stage. Previous observational studies can now be reassessed in the light of recent developments and more rational advice can be given on diet and lifestyle issues.

Protein metabolism

Protein in the diet comes from meat, fish, eggs, dairy products, pulses and nuts. All proteins are made up of amino acids. When proteins are eaten, they are broken down in the stomach firstly into peptides by the enzyme pepsin, and then into amino acids by enzymes secreted from the pancreas into the small intestine. Two forms of amino acid exist: essential and non-essential amino acids. The body can make its own non-essential amino acids but essential amino acids are obtained from the diet from either animal protein or a combination of plant proteins. The amino acids absorbed from the digestive tract are metabolised by the liver and can be used to make new proteins that make up cells. Alternatively certain amino acids can be converted into glucose. This is essential for maintaining blood glucose levels during periods of low carbohydrate consumption, or the early stages of starvation before fat utilisation has been fully activated, for example, overnight.

Fat metabolism

Dietary fat is a complex mixture of triacylglycerols, previously referred to as triglycerides (TGs), phospholipids (PLs), and sterol esters derived from the cells of animal adipose (fatty) tissue or plant oils. Fat is virtually insoluble in water, so it must first be emulsified to be made available for enzymic digestion. This is accomplished in the duodenum, where dietary fat is mixed with bile fluid secreted by the gall bladder in response to a fat-rich meal. The bile fluid contains bile salts and lecithin which act as detergents to disperse and emulsify the fat and oil-soluble vitamins A, D, E, K and the carotenoids into mixed micelles, which are then acted upon by the enzymes of the alkaline pancreatic secretion. Different enzymes then digest the TGs, PLs and cholesterol esters found in animal food fats. The digestion products are then absorbed into the cells of the mucosal wall which are called enterocytes, where they may be resynthesised back into the starting materials, and eventually transported into the blood for use as energy or transported to the liver for further processing, or stored in the adipose tissue.

Once in the blood, fat and cholesterol can be used by all of the cells in the body. Fats and cholesterol are major constituents of cell membranes, and like proteins they are vitally important for health. Fat and carbohydrate metabolism are very closely linked under the influence of the hormones insulin and glucagon. Sterols from plant fats are not metabolised, so true vegans must derive their cholesterol from synthesis in the liver. Chapter 5 explains in detail which fats are good and which are bad for our health, and how they are transported around the body in different lipoprotein complexes.

Carbohydrate metabolism

The carbohydrates we eat are mainly derived from plants, although meat contains a small amount of animal starch called glycogen. Foods rich in carbohydrates include rice, bread, pasta and potatoes; they contain starch, which is digested to yield glucose. Pure sugar from sugar cane and sugar beet is sucrose which is digested to yield glucose and fructose, the sugar found in most sweet fruits. Many soft or fizzy drinks are also rich in sucrose but this is increasingly being replaced by high fructose corn syrup. Beer contains sugars from malted barley.

All the forms of carbohydrate consumed are eventually converted in our bodies to glucose. Glucose is the form of sugar found in the blood and is what medical doctors and scientists refer to as blood sugar. This is a major source of energy for the cells in our bodies. After a meal containing carbohydrate, the amount of glucose in the blood increases; the degree of increase depends upon the type and the amount of carbohydrate consumed. The glucose released from digestion will either be used immediately to provide energy or stored for the future. Some glucose is converted to glycogen (a glucose polymer similar to plant starch), which is stored in the liver and muscles. Glycogen is a form of carbohydrate that can be used quickly by the body when it needs energy for high intensity activity like sprinting. The remaining excess glucose is turned into fat and deposited in the adipose (fatty) tissue. Under normal conditions we get fatter, but if we are under stress that fat can be deposited on our artery walls and around the midriff,[3] leading to an increased risk of heart disease. These glucose storage mechanisms are controlled by the hormone insulin.

When food was scarce 100,000 years ago, the human digestive system evolved and still functions to this day to extract the maximum nutrient from a poor diet. Since we no longer live in a nutrient-poor environment, after eating a high carbohydrate (sugar-rich) diet, the body is flooded with glucose. This results in a rise in the level of the hormone insulin secreted from the

---

[3] Abdominal obesity is discussed in detail in Chapters 8 and 9.

pancreas and released into the blood stream. This has the effect of lowering the blood sugar level, usually to a level lower than before the sugar was eaten (see Figure 1). This low blood sugar induces a craving for more sugar. This cycle can, if not controlled by eating a low or complex carbohydrate diet, leads to a pre-diabetic state and can increase the risk of obesity, cancer and heart disease, explained in more detail later.

Insulin is essential for the maintenance of a healthy blood sugar level. Insulin is a hormone secreted by the pancreas, in response to a rise in blood glucose. Insulin regulates the amount of glucose in our blood by stimulating cellular uptake and the storage of any excess as glycogen and body fat.

How insulin controls carbohydrate and lipid metabolism

The single most important factor in controlling carbohydrate metabolism and fat utilisation and storage is the hormone insulin. Insulin also activates an enzyme that promotes the transport of fatty acids, the products of fat digestion and biosynthesis, in the blood into adipose cells for storage as fat. Insulin also prevents the breakdown of previously stored fat for energy use and stimulates the production of cholesterol in the liver.

After eating a meal high in carbohydrates, there is an initial blood sugar increase, as glucose is released by the digestive system. After a while, the effect of insulin suppresses our blood sugar level, often to a level lower than before the carbohydrate was eaten (see Figure 1). Approximately 30 minutes

17

after a meal rich in carbohydrates, blood sugar peaks. Low blood sugar (hypoglycaemia) is seen at approximately 60 minutes after a carbohydrate-rich meal and blood sugar can remain at abnormally low levels for about two hours. This is responsible for the lethargic sleepy feelings experienced after large meals, and later can cause cravings for more carbohydrate-rich food in an attempt to raise the blood sugar and its associated, though short-lived, feelings of well-being. This is particularly apparent after consuming sugar-rich soft drinks and sweets.

With age we become less able to deal with large changes in blood sugar levels and the subsequent insulin peaks, and older people become sleepy after carbohydrate-rich meals. Unfit people are also less capable of stabilising their blood sugar because their muscles do not demand as much sugar as those of active people.

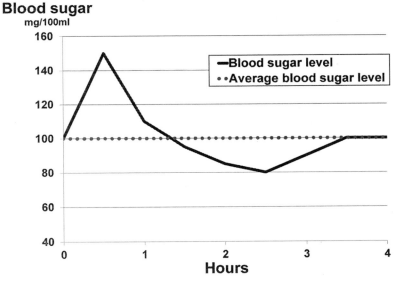

Figure 1 **The rise and fall in blood sugar before and after a carbohydrate rich meal.**

The muscles of an active person, irrespective of age, absorb more sugar for the production of glycogen than those of inactive individuals, and hence less glucose is available for fat deposition in active individuals.

Insulin plays a major role in body fat deposition. If the amount of insulin released into the blood can be reduced, then the amount of fat deposited around the body can be limited. The amount of insulin released into the blood depends on the amount of glucose absorbed from digestion. By consuming fewer refined carbohydrates, the most readily available sources of dietary glucose, less insulin is secreted and less body fat deposited.

People on a persistently high carbohydrate diet, particularly the overweight and the obese, often secrete excessive quantities of insulin, which only compounds their problems. In the long term, this can lead to a condition called insulin resistance, where the cells in the body do not respond to insulin in the way that they should. Insulin receptors on the surface of the cells are prevented from stimulating the absorption of glucose. As a result the cells are starved of energy. This is one reason why some overweight people suffer from fatigue and are always hungry. Since insulin is not stimulating the transport of glucose into cells, it transfers more and more glucose into stored body fat.

Persistently high blood insulin, with the cells of the body not responding properly to its effects, will ultimately result in what is known as hyperinsulinaemia. In many cases this is followed by the development of diabetes Type 2. Diabetes can lead to an increased risk of heart disease and has long-term adverse effects upon the eyes, kidneys, skin, nervous system and peripheral blood circulation. The main cause of this is a diet high in sugar and refined carbohydrates.

Glucagon, the starvation hormone

Glucagon is another of the body's hormones secreted by the pancreas and is released into the blood after a protein-rich meal or during starvation. Glucagon induces the release of previously stored body fat, allowing the tissues to derive energy from body fat. Once the glucagon level is raised, it will remain so for some time and continue to stimulate our body to burn fat. This hormone also inhibits the first enzyme in the pathway of fatty acid biosynthesis; this reduces the build-up of body fat. Carbohydrate-rich meals will suppress glucagon secretion, and increase insulin secretion, which leads to fat storage. This basic knowledge is the underlying theory upon which several popular, successful low carbohydrate weight loss books are based, such as *Sugar Busters*, *The Atkins New Diet Revolution*, *The Stone-Age Diet* and the *CSIRO Total Wellbeing Diet*.

The human body: designed to survive starvation, not excessive eating

There is a great deal of relevance in how our body is designed to cope with periods of starvation, even though in the modern Western world, starvation is rarely experienced. The important fact to appreciate is that our bodies are capable of withstanding prolonged periods of starvation, but today the abundance of food overwhelms our bodies, leading to obesity and related diseases.

Certain people have what is known as a thrifty metabolism. This involves the very efficient use of available dietary calories, even during periods of starvation. This leads to food calories being stored as fat in the adipose tissue when food is readily available. These stores of body fat will then be available to be used as energy during any subsequent periods of starvation.

An example of such a metabolism can be seen today in the Polynesian populations. Obesity [8], heart disease [9] and diabetes [10] have reached epidemic proportions within these populations. This problem has arisen as a result of the consumption of refined foods high in carbohydrates and calories in general, with no intervening periods of starvation. The presence of this phenomenon in a mixed population will result in wide variations in weight loss or gain when the same diets are eaten. It would seem, therefore, that people with more efficient energy metabolism are more at risk of obesity when consuming modern junk food diets.

Our bodies use the food we eat very efficiently. Excess calories are quickly turned into body fat, which is a store of energy to be used when food is scarce. Problems arise due to over consumption of refined foods high in carbohydrates with no intervening periods of starvation. Body fat is deposited but not metabolised thanks to the presence of excess carbohydrate.

Human responses to starvation

A healthy adult is capable of withstanding a 40 day fast, as long as water is available. Our ability to withstand starvation is best understood by thinking of our body as a food reserve which we can use as an energy source in times of starvation. These fuel reserves consist of fat in our adipose tissue, glycogen in our liver and muscles and protein in our muscles and organs. These fuel reserves are used at differing rates and at different times during starvation to prevent low blood glucose and catastrophic muscle wasting as a result of excessive protein breakdown.

21

Table 1 **Fuel reserves of an average 70kg man (154lb) in kilocalories**

Fat	100000
Protein	25000
Glucose	40
Glycogen	
– muscles	400
– liver	200

Low blood glucose can lead to faintness, lethargy, clumsiness and even coma, and so the body has intricate methods of avoiding low blood glucose and the associated mental and physical impairments.

Table 1 shows the fuel reserves of an average 70kg man (154lb) in kilocalories (seen on food packaging as kcal). This is an approximate total of 125,640 kilocalories of fuel contained within the body of an average (not overweight) man. Significant amounts of this fuel supply can be used during periods of starvation. Protein loss must be minimised. So, from the table, we can see that we could survive approximately 50 days utilising the calories from fat alone, assuming 2,000 calories are used per day. Note that the body's carbohydrate store is extremely limited and as a result, utilisation is controlled very stringently (see Figures 2 and 3). Note the 200-fold difference in the scale of Figures 2 and 3. These figures represent data for an average 70kg man. An overweight individual would have correspondingly more reserves and a capacity to survive much longer periods of starvation. The very slow breakdown of protein is necessary to allow muscles to continue working, and later in starvation to maintain a basal level of glucose production for brain and red blood cell metabolism. This is strikingly demonstrated in Figure 2, which shows what happens when the protein and fat fuel reserves of a 70kg man are utilised over a 40-day period of starvation [11].

Carbohydrate metabolism is even more stringently controlled. It can be seen in Figure 3 that there is a 44% loss over the first night, but then there is little or no change in the body's carbohydrate reserve. The biggest changes are seen in the body's fat reserves, reflecting their role as the major energy store. The fact that the body switches to utilising body fat as a source of energy during starvation is the basis of several modern, low carbohydrate diet regimes. Here, we outline the typical changes in the body that happen during starvation, as this sheds light on the efficacy of many modern diets.

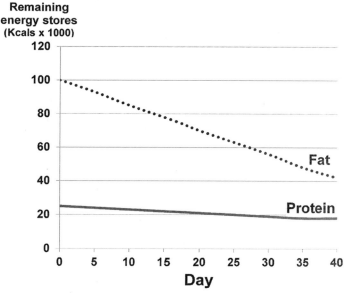

Figure 2 The loss of fat and protein energy reserves over 40 days of total starvation in a 70kg man.

Changes in the body's metabolism during starvation

On the first day of starvation, the blood glucose levels remain unchanged as we use the remaining glucose available from the gut. The second phase of starvation occurs at night (during sleep) and involves the stores of liver glycogen being broken down in an attempt to maintain the blood glucose level. During the early hours of the next morning, the body reduces glycogen breakdown and begins to breakdown the muscle tissue protein. Usually only about 1% of the muscle tissue will be broken down and if food is eaten in the morning, no ill effects will be felt from this process.

If starvation continues, however, protein breakdown continues at a low rate in order to maintain blood glucose levels, and body fat is broken down into fatty acids and glycerol at a steady rate continuously throughout starvation. The fatty acids

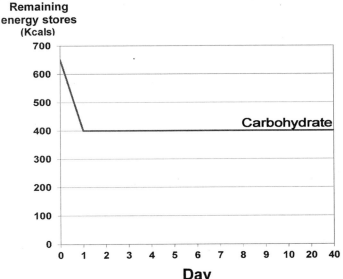

Figure 3 The utilisation of carbohydrate over a 40-day period of total starvation in a 70kg man.

are transported to the liver, where they are converted into ketones which serve as low molecular weight, water-soluble sources of energy. The ketones are then transported to the muscles and organs, particularly the brain, to be used as an energy source. Unlike fatty acids which can be toxic at high concentrations, ketone levels in the blood can rise 100-fold, without any toxic side effects, following starvation. During this stage of starvation the brain will switch from a 100% to a 25% glucose requirement, the remaining energy (75%) being supplied as ketones and amino acids. In non-exercising starving subjects, the switch to a ketogenic metabolism takes about a week to become fully active. This induction period was also experienced in the late 1800s by Arctic explorers, who switched to the high fat diets of the traditional Inuit, and forms the basis for the Atkins-type diets, which trick the body into responding to a low carbohydrate diet in the same way it would if we were starving. Hence body fat is broken down and we get slimmer without drastically depleting the body's reserves of muscle protein and glycogen.

Another crucial feature of low carbohydrate/high fat diets is that the blood glucose level is adequately maintained. This is carried out by the process of gluconeogenesis (making new glucose) from non-carbohydrate precursors, mainly proteins. Unlike the breakdown of starch to glucose the process requires energy since 100g of protein only yields 57g of glucose. This process is fuelled by increased fat oxidation, since protein must be conserved under these conditions. Furthermore, high fat diets increase energy loss by activating the process of thermogenesis where metabolic energy is released as heat to maintain the body temperature, which is a useful feature if you are living in an igloo on Arctic sea ice and relying on a diet of oily fish and seal meat and blubber. Detailed diaries and reports from early explorers in the Arctic regions reveal the remarkable properties of these diets which were capable of sustaining the Inuit and their Western guests through many months of extreme physical endurance with no apparent ill effects on the return to 'civilisation'. Of particular note was the lack of scurvy despite the supposed low vitamin C in their diets. In addition, the myth of high protein Inuit diets was exposed, as they were found to consume 80–85% fat, 5–15% protein and 3–5% carbohydrate. Their folk history also stressed the dangers of a high lean meat diet, and explorers noted that, when food was short, they always gave lean meat to the dog teams and reserved the fatty cuts for themselves. When the adventurers returned, there was a flurry of interest and a rush to reproduce the results in laboratories. Several short-term studies revealed that the switch from normal high carbohydrate diets to high fat regimes resulted in the very opposite effects to those seen with traditional Inuit diets.

Subjects suffered debilitating effects with headaches, lassitude and the inability to perform demanding physical tasks. One such study, aimed at assessing the use of pemmican (dried meat and fat) as lightweight emergency food for troops in the Second World War, failed at the first hurdle and was aborted after only three days when the troops became unable to perform their allotted physical tasks [12]. If the researchers had had access to the diaries of those explorers in the previous century, they would have learned that this switch from a high carbohydrate to a high fat diet involved a transient drop in well-being and energy for around two weeks [13]. Following this period, normal activities could be resumed with no ill effects. Moreover, several other studies reporting the ill effects of high fat diets were also short-term and did not take into account crucial losses of dietary minerals associated with inappropriate cooking techniques, such as boiling and discarding the mineral-rich cooking water. These phenomena have now been reassessed in carefully designed

26

metabolic experiments with both trained and untrained human subjects [14]. Both groups experienced a lag in performance in the first couple of weeks following carbohydrate restriction, after which time full endurance performance was restored. These are some of very few studies, among the many thousands of dietary investigations, which address the crucial link between dietary fat utilisation and exercise. It should be noted that high fat diets will not sustain vigorous anaerobic exercise such as sprinting and weightlifting because of rapid muscle glycogen depletion and onset of exhaustion.

Inadequate emergency diets high in carbohydrate fed to starving children may be more damaging, in the short term, than eating no food at all, if that food is low in protein and fat, and rich in carbohydrate. A small amount of carbohydrate, as little as 50g a day, not enough to supply the daily calorie needs, can stop the body utilising fat as an energy source and force it to breakdown protein to maintain the blood glucose supply, stimulating the destruction of muscles and other tissues. The devastating results of partial starvation have been seen in some of the food aid programs to the African sub-continent where starving children were given insufficient calories, supplied as low fat/protein, high carbohydrate food, which resulted in excess muscle wasting and massive weight loss, catastrophic protein deficiency and death.

We propose that the underlying metabolic processes will be almost identical in cachexia (tissue wasting) and partial starvation. Cachexia is responsible for 40% of all cancer deaths. In many cancer patients, the tumour tissue will be consuming sugar at a greater rate that it can be supplied in the diet, thus switching on the ultimately fatal process of muscle wastage. At the same time, the tumour secretes factors that will stimulate fat metabolism in the patient, thus enabling all of the carbohydrates to be channelled to the cancer, whilst the host survives temporarily on the mobilised body fat. Although no clinical trials have been carried out to test this hypothesis, it is possible that an Atkins-type diet may be beneficial to cachexic patients in that they will be provided with adequate calories in the form of fat and protein, but insufficient carbohydrate to switch on excessive protein breakdown and muscle wastage, and at the same time reducing tumour growth by carbohydrate restriction.

Sources of dietary sugar

Choice of carbohydrate to maintain a healthy insulin level

Sugar contained in processed food is usually in the form of high fructose corn syrup or sucrose. Other carbohydrates include lactose in milk and starch in plants and glycogen in meat. Refined carbohydrates (starches) in white flour are converted to glucose very quickly by our digestive systems and raise blood glucose levels almost as rapidly as pure sugars.

The term complex carbohydrate is now used to describe mixtures of starch and dietary fibre polysaccharides which are not broken down by human digestive enzymes. The fibres can be divided into two categories; soluble and insoluble. Soluble fibres can form a viscous solution in the small intestine which slows down the release and uptake of glucose. Foods rich in soluble fibres include apples, porridge and legumes. Insoluble fibre such as cellulose bulks up the gut contents and limits access of the digestive enzymes to the starch. The starch in unrefined brown flour in whole grain breads and pasta and brown rice is digested much more slowly due to the presence of complex carbohydrate and does not cause the peaks and troughs of insulin production that follow the consumption of refined carbohydrates. Some complex carbohydrates can be converted into glucose, but at a reduced rate. Their consumption can help prevent insulin overproduction and its associated problems. Another form of complex carbohydrate known as resistant starch is not broken down to glucose by the enzymes of the small intestine. It reaches the colon and is consumed by the resident bacteria which generate butyric acid. The beneficial effects of dietary resistant starch are explained in Chapter 3. Also, different sugars vary in the speed at which they enter our blood stream. Eating glucose will allow the most sugar into the blood followed by fructose (fruit sugar), sucrose and lactose. Different forms of a particular food can also lead to different blood sugar levels.

The amount of sugar obtained from a particular food depends on the amount of different carbohydrates within that food. The amount of sugar released from rice depends on the proportion of the two main types of starch found in rice: amylose and amylopectin. Rice with more amylopectin will release more glucose into the blood when compared with rice rich in amylose, because amylopectin is digested more rapidly than amylose [15]. For example, Basmati rice contains a high proportion of amylose and is therefore a good source of slow-release calories.

Different types of pasta also release different amounts of sugar; for example, macaroni releases more than spaghetti [16]. Even within a variety of pasta such as linguine, a different thickness will result in differing amounts of sugar being released. Thin linguine allows more sugar to be released into the blood than thick linguine as a consequence of the greater surface area of the thin linguine, as greater surface area means faster digestion and release of sugars to raise blood glucose levels.

29

How food preparation affects sugar use

Starch exists as large granules in carbohydrate foods. Disruption of these granules by heating, grinding, rolling, pressing and chewing increases the amount of sugar and the rate at which it is released into the blood. This is a consequence of the increased surface area of the food and hence the increased rate of digestion in the intestine. The way in which food is prepared can alter the amount of sugar released into the blood. For example, 25% more sugar is released from potato when it is mashed before eating, when compared to cutting it into chips [17]. Eating whole apples releases less sugar into the blood than apple puree, which in turn releases less sugar than drinking apple juice [18]. This idea can be applied to all fruit and vegetables, and to other sources of nutrients; for example, more protein will be released from minced beef than from steak.

The less manipulated or refined a food product is, the less sugar is released when it is digested. The cooking method affects sugar release beyond the effects of mashing or pureeing food. For example, in uncooked potato the starch granules are resistant to digestion, but when potato is cooked, the starch granules are disrupted and become readily digestible and will lead to rapid increases in the blood sugar levels. When cooking a food like potato, the heat used, the amount of water and the length of cooking time all have significant effects on sugar release [18]. Therefore the more a starch-containing food is heated, moisturised and ground, the more easily it will be digested, releasing its sugar into the small intestine.

Glycaemic load and glycaemic index

Glycaemic load (GL) refers to the total glucose releasing capacity of the food. This is different from the glycaemic index (GI) which measures the rate at which sugar is released into the blood over a given time period when a particular food is eaten. Many people and dietary plans use the GI as a guide to control of sugar consumption. This may not be the best method to use. The GL may give a more accurate representation for dietary purposes. For example, water melon has a high GI. This means that when water melon is eaten, the sugar it contains is released very rapidly (high GI), but it does not actually contain a great deal of sugar (low GL). High GI water melon can therefore be a good dietary aid. Conversely, high GI foods rich in refined sugar and/or starch such as fizzy drinks, cakes and confectionery, make a major contribution to the GL and should be avoided on calorie-controlled diets. The GI may be more relevant in diseases such as diabetes, where rapid uptake of available sugar can be harmful.

The World Health Organisation (WHO) now recommends that no more than 5% of our total calorific intake should come from sugar. This refers to the total sugar intake from processed foods (biscuits and cakes etc) as well as that added to tea, coffee, breakfast cereals and desserts, for example. Most people in developed countries consume more than this. Direct comparisons are difficult to make, but The United States Department of Agriculture (USDA) data for 2000 quote US sugar consumption values of 19% of total calories consumed. The average sugar consumption between April 2004 and December 2006 in the UK was 14.4% [19]. We consume a diet high in sugars, fats and salt, mainly as a result of the amount of fast food and processed food in our modern diet. We can reduce the amount of sugar that we add to our tea, coffee, breakfast cereal and so on, and we can also reduce the amount of sugar we consume by reducing the amount of pre-prepared foods we eat. Most if not all of these products contain labels indicating the amount of sugar in that particular product, usually measured in g per 100g of solid product or

100ml of liquid. Many fizzy drinks contain as much as 18% sugar. Whilst this is important and tells us the amount of sugar consumed, it does not indicate the proportion of the daily 5% accounted for by this amount of sugar. The average American consumes 2,750 calories per day, compared with the 2,200 calories recommended for most children, teenage girls, active women, and sedentary men.

If this is taken as a guide along with the WHO recommendation to consume 5% of the daily calories as sugar, then children can safely eat 110 calories of added sugar per day. One gram of sugar contains approximately 4 calories, so 27.5g of sugar contains 110 calories. Children should therefore eat no more than 27.5g of added sugar per day to be within the WHO recommendations. The consumption of a 330ml can of cola will deliver between 30-40g of sugar well above the WHO recommendation. Given that on average we should consume no more than 27.5g of added sugar per day, it is useful to look at where we get this sugar from and which readily available foods contain the most and least added sugar. The nature of the added sugar should also be ascertained as the potentially harmful high fructose syrup replaces sucrose in more and more food and drink products.

3   Sugar: a drug and a poison?

Recent research has revealed that addiction to sugar
involves pathways in the brain which are identical to
those associated with hard drug addiction, and
highlights the difficulties in operating successful anti-
obesity programmes. We now expand on this and some
of the many negative effects that high blood sugar can
have on our health.

We also reveal how food processing and preparation
affect the amount of glucose released from food. The
reasons why some carbohydrates are better than others
are discussed with reference to resistant starch and the
replacement of sugar with high fructose corn syrup in
many processed foods and drinks. In addition, the
politics and economics behind the junk food epidemic
are discussed.

Introduction

In many cultures, with the possible exception of the traditional
Inuit, sugar has become a ubiquitous source of pleasure and self-
indulgence. Research in the new millennium has shown why
many of us are hooked on sugar. There is now compelling
evidence that sugar can alter our brain chemistry by the same
biochemical mechanisms that drive the addiction to hard drugs
such as cocaine and heroin, and to a lesser extent, nicotine and
alcohol. Furthermore, this effect is reinforced by the presence of
fat and salt in highly palatable sugar-rich junk foods.

33

Sugar and drug addiction: the role of dopamine

Addiction to any substance or process involves a de-sensitisation of the 'reward circuits' in the brain caused by overconsumption of the stimulant. This causes the addict to consume even more to compensate for the lack of pleasurable response that occurred initially. The pursuit of pleasure from food, drugs and sex (and probably rock and roll!) involves the release of the neuro-transmitter dopamine in the brain, which then binds to receptors in the pleasure centres of the brain. In healthy animals and humans this then completes the reward circuitry and reduces the craving for further gratification, i.e. the stimulant is no longer required. In addicts, the circuit is not completed as the dopamine receptors become de-sensitised. Recent ground-breaking research has shown that there are genetic determinants in obesity where people are born with an innate love of eating sugar-rich foods. This leads to overeating and a dulling of the reward circuitry as in chronic alcohol or substance abuse. An additional cause of obesity results from inherited defects in the DRD2 and DRD4 dopamine receptor genes, which results in the need to eat more, to get an adequate reward [21]. This work has been supported in animal feeding studies [22–24].

Compulsive eating in obese but not lean rats was associated with down-regulation of the D2R dopamine receptors. When these receptors were artificially reduced in the brains of healthy, lean rats, the effects were dramatic. The treated rats immediately gorged on junk foods to the extent of tolerating electric shocks and ignored normal rat food where no painful stimulus was involved. When fed from the outset on normal rat food, these treated animals did not respond by overeating. The development of obesity in rats and probably humans must therefore involve a combination of junk food and defects in the reward circuitry. This latest research highlights the problems behind the current obesity epidemic fuelled by the junk food industry. If fast food stimulates the same behaviour as that caused by hard drugs, then perhaps the industry should be subject to more stringent regulations.

How can we say that sugar is a poison? It is true that blood sugar is essential for health, but the consumption of sugar is not. Some authorities would have us believe that sugar consumption is harmless. This is not true. A massive and uncontrolled expansion of the fast food industry has helped fuel the huge rise in sugar content of the Western diet. One should not be misled by recent publicity about sugar consumption going down in the US. This decrease refers only to sucrose consumption, i.e. the sugar added to food at home. Since 1980 the use of high fructose syrup as a sucrose replacement in processed foods has expanded at an unprecedented rate which appears to mirror the increase in obesity in the US.

In 2000, the average American consumed an astounding 2 to 3lb of added sugar per week in their diet (USDA Economic Research Service), and Britain is not far behind with a Defra report indicating a consumption of 1.9lb per week in 2006 [20]. This is an average US consumption of 5,600 calories per week from sugar alone, and is almost three days' worth of total calories every week with no nutritional value and the potential to gain at least 1lb of body fat per week! The same USDA study also revealed that cane/beet sugar consumption had dropped by 33% since 1950, from 88% of the total sugar calories to 43%. This deficit has been more than filled by the corn sweeteners, and in particular, high fructose syrup. The consumption of which increased 10 fold by 2000 (Figure 4).

35

This is an extremely worrying state of affairs as the literature is full of studies on the negative association of high fructose with blood urate, inflammation, hypertension, insulin resistance, Syndrome X and its symptom obesity, dislipidaemia (elevated blood lipids) and CVD [25]. Children are particularly at risk thanks to their high consumption of fizzy drinks and convenience foods, which are increasingly sweetened with high fructose syrups which are not naturally present in foods at such high concentrations.

The data (see figure 4) suggests a direct link between the consumption of high fructose corn syrup and the obesity epidemic with the obesity curve inflection in 1977 mirroring the increase in consumption of corn syrup.

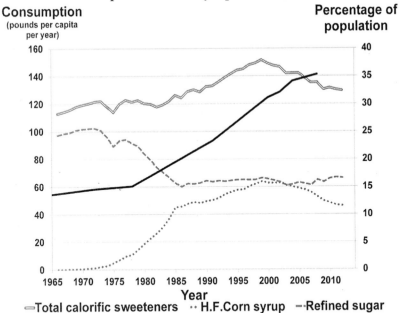

Figure 4 US consumption of total and component caloric sweetners since 1965.

To spell this out, our great grand-parents consumed 5lb of sugar in a year, with much lower risks of sugar-related diseases.

Health hazards associated with excessive fructose intake

Early dietary experiments with fructose were associated with the consumption of fruit and vegetables and indicated that a modest daily consumption of fructose of 16–20g improved the control of blood glucose levels. This led health and medical practitioners to encourage its use as a replacement for glucose and sucrose in diabetic diets. The widespread use of high fructose corn syrup (HFCS) as a replacement for sucrose in soft drinks and processed foods since the 1970s has resulted in a fivefold increase in uptake to 85–100g/day in the US and Europe.

Nutritional properties of fructose

All sugars are not equivalent to glucose in terms of energy release or fat accumulation, and humans have a limited capacity to deal with high intakes of fructose. Dietary fructose enters the liver and interferes with the normal process of blood sugar control by glucose. It is rapidly metabolised to glucose precursors but more importantly to fatty acid and TG precursors, ultimately leading to insulin resistance and obesity. The health outcomes from excessive fructose consumption are summarised below:

- Interference with the control of energy metabolism in the liver.

- It is converted to glucose in the liver but does not stimulate insulin synthesis in the pancreas, leading to:

- A reduction in leptin synthesis and loss of appetite suppression.

- It provides substrates for a massive increase in fatty acid and TG synthesis in the liver. This in turn leads to:

- Increased liver and serum TG, liver enlargement and hepatic steatosis (fatty liver), and overproduction of VLDL particles. This metabolic state culminates in:

- Obesity

- Metabolic syndrome and finally Type 2 diabetes.

- Stimulation of TG synthesis also leads to lipid peroxidation and general oxidative stress which can initiate cancers and CVD.

- Recent research has shown that fructose also accelerates cancer cell division by stimulating DNA synthesis.

The above list supports the warning to avoid all drinks and processed foods containing HFCS.

In conclusion, sugar intake has risen drastically without any changes in the body's ability to dispose of or use the sugar we eat. In other words, we would have to increase our exercise regimes to an impossible level to use all those extra calories we take in. Some people are lucky enough to be able to burn off these calories as heat through a process termed Non Exercise Activity Thermogenesis (NEAT), which is explained in more detail in Chapter 8.

It is possible to find over 100 different ways in which sugar can damage the human body; in the following section, we highlight those that we consider the most important.

Sugar and the immune system

It is essential for good health to maintain a strong immune system, and a good diet and exercise are crucial for this. The immune system requires the complex interaction of a number of cells and compounds within the body. These components work together to kill bacteria and viruses.

White blood cells are a critical component of our immune system. Unfortunately, eating sugar makes white blood cells considerably less effective in their protective role. For example, eating or drinking approximately 100g of sugar, the equivalent of two cans of cola (660ml), can reduce the ability of the white blood cells to kill germs by 40%. This effect starts less than 30 minutes after ingestion and may last for up to five hours [26]. In contrast, eating complex carbohydrates has no apparent ill effect on the immune system. It has also been shown that a high blood glucose level of 120mg/ml, a blood sugar level not uncommon in the Western world, reduces the ability of white blood cells to fight infection by 75%.

White blood cells need relatively large amounts of vitamin C to work effectively (about 50 times the amount found in the blood). When blood glucose is high, vitamin C uptake from the blood is reduced. This occurs because glucose is absorbed by these cells in the same way as vitamin C. These two molecules compete for the same point of entry into the white blood cells.

Sugar and kidney damage

Persistently high blood glucose can damage to the membranes of the kidney [27]. Glucose is known to react with proteins in the lining of capillaries, resulting in loss of elasticity and increased fragility. This allows protein that would normally stay in the blood to pass into the urine. If damage to the membranes continues, kidney failure may result. This is most commonly seen in diabetics, who have persistently high blood glucose.

Sugar and cardiovascular disease (atherosclerosis)

The stages in cardiovascular disease

Cardiovascular disease (CVD) or atherosclerosis is the commonest cause of death in the developed world. Heart attacks and most strokes are the end-points of degenerative changes caused by atherosclerosis. This disease is characterised by a thickening of the artery wall that develops in the inner coat or intima. Three stages are involved in the progressive obstruction of the artery:

1. Formation of raised yellow fatty streaks characterised by lipid-rich foam cells derived from macrophages and smooth muscle cells. Fatty streaks, which have been seen even in babies on Western sugar/fat-rich diets, are probably precursors of the next stage.

2. Fibrous plaques which are raised, round lesions, off-white and up to 1cm in diameter. They consist of a fibrous cap of mainly smooth muscle cells and connective tissue (collagen), with macrophages, more smooth muscle cells and T-lymphocytes beneath. Deeper layers contain dead, necrotic cells, extra-cellular lipids and cholesterol crystals. The fibrous plaques can progress to the final stage of arterial obstruction.

3. The complicated plaque, which is the most dangerous stage, is unstable due to further necrosis causing release of degradative protease enzymes, calcium deposition, bleeding and minor thrombosis. Major thrombosis leading to complete arterial blockage occurs when the plaque ruptures releasing its noxious contents into the blood stream. These products stimulate platelet aggregation at the ruptured plaque site to form a large blood clot. Such clots in the large arteries to the heart will cause a heart attack. In the brain arteries they will cause a stroke.

Sugar raises the insulin level in the blood leading to increased TG [28]. Higher levels of TGs in the blood raise the risk of heart disease [29].

Regular consumption of high carbohydrate foods and a resultant persistently high insulin level can result in a condition called insulin resistance. If we are insulin resistant, the insulin we produce is less effective at getting sugar in our blood to our cells. As a result, sugar remains in the blood. This can lead to diabetes and/or Syndrome X (metabolic syndrome), both of which raise the risk of heart disease [30]. Syndrome X is a cluster of risk factors that include high levels of insulin, TGs, low high density lipoprotein (HDL) and high low density lipoprotein (LDL) in the blood, with increased blood pressure. Some 47 million Americans have been diagnosed with Syndrome X. The terms HDL and LDL refer to the lipoprotein complexes that transport cholesterol in the blood stream [31]. HDL particles are commonly referred to as 'good' cholesterol and transport cholesterol to the liver where it is converted to bile acids and secreted into the small intestine. LDL particles or 'bad' cholesterol are lipid rich and contain lipoprotein (a), which can cause them to stick to artery walls and initiate plaque formation and in particular it is the small oxidised forms

41

of LDL which are the major risk factor. This situation was exacerbated in the US in 1977, when the US Public Health recommendations suggested a lowering of fat intake to less than 30% of total calories, to lower the incidence of CHD. The Food and Drug Administration (FDA) responded and recommended high carbohydrate diets which were subsequently found to contribute to changed blood lipid patterns, characteristic of an increased risk of heart disease.

Recent research has indicated that there is a relationship between high carbohydrate diets and heart disease in middle-aged women [19, 32]. The studies suggest that inflammation in the arteries, caused by the consumption of carbohydrates, may be responsible. Inflammation can stimulate white blood cells to attack fatty deposits lining the arteries. This can cause fragments to break off and clog the arteries. In advanced cases, this may trigger a full-fledged heart attack or stroke. Since everyone is familiar with the reference to LDL as 'bad' cholesterol, it should be stressed that this is an over-simplification. Low density lipoprotein particles only become a risk factor following inflammation when they become oxidised by free radicals and are subsequently taken up by macrophages and smooth muscle cells to form lipid overloaded foam cells (see Appendix for further details).

Sugar and free radical formation in the blood stream

Free radicals are highly reactive, unstable molecules produced by the white blood cells that can perform beneficial tasks such as aiding in the destruction of microorganisms and cancer cells. Inappropriate or excessive free radical formation can result in the attack on biological molecules that damage protein, lipids and DNA in the body under conditions known as oxidative stress.

High blood sugar levels can activate cellular enzymes that produce free radicals in the blood [33]. This can lead to damage in the kidney, eye and heart tissues as well as blood vessel contraction, reduced blood flow and increased blood pressure. Free radicals have also been implicated in a number of diseases including many cancers, Alzheimer's disease, arthritis and asthma [34–37].

Sugar and cancer

In the second half of the 20th century, one trillion dollars was expended on the development of chemotherapy for cancer treatment. Little effort was spent on the potential of dietary intervention, even though it has been known since 1931 that the metabolism of tumour cells is very different from that of healthy cells with respect to sugar consumption.

Basically, tumour cells require glucose as an energy source and will not survive without it. Otto Warburg won the Nobel Prize for Science for this work. The crux of Warburg's Nobel thesis was that tumours use glucose as an energy supply just as normal healthy cells do, but they extract the energy in a different way, without using oxygen [38]. This is not efficient and the tumour only gets about 5% of the available energy from the glucose. By extracting only 5% of the available energy, the tumour is wasting energy. So, in order to survive, the tumour needs ten times more sugar than healthy cells require, and it will not survive without this extra sugar.

Following on from this important work in the early 1940s, scientists demonstrated that animals with chemically induced cancer survived longer when starved than those on an unrestricted diet. More recent studies suggest that a diet with a high glycaemic

43

load (high sugar content) may increase the risk of colorectal cancer [39] and breast cancer in women [40], in addition to many chronic diseases.

A mouse model for brain cancer has recently been developed and has shown that ketogenic (low carbohydrate) diets cause spectacular tumour regression. As in humans, the healthy mouse brain appears to be able to use ketones as a substitute energy source and the tumours regress and die due to the lack of dietary glucose. This diet appears to act by preventing the tumours from stimulating the mouse tissues to degrade their protein to form glucose to feed the tumours. In other words, this means that the mice do not become cachexic (see below). We believe that this study offers very exciting possibilities, in the first instance, for the non-invasive treatment of brain cancer, and ultimately for the treatment of all cancers [41].

To ensure growth, tumour cells absorb a lot of sugar. They do this by secreting insulin, which binds to insulin receptors on their own cell membranes (tumour cells have approximately ten times more insulin receptors than normal cells). Insulin stimulates cells to take up glucose and as tumour cells secrete insulin and have more receptors, they absorb more of the blood glucose than normal cells. This is an adaptation of the tumour cells in response to their inefficient use of glucose, and without it the tumours would not obtain enough energy for survival.

Tumour cells also secrete an insulin-like growth factor, and have approximately ten times more insulin-like growth factor receptors than normal cells. In addition to ten times more glucose transporters, these characteristics allow tumour cell increased growth to out-compete healthy cells for available glucose [42].

44

If you deprive a tumour of sugar by eating little or no carbohydrate, less glucose will enter the blood and less sugar will be available for the tumour to use as energy. Another way of depriving tumour cells of glucose involves eating vegetables like avocados, which contain an unusual sugar called mannoheptulose that can block excess glucose receptors on the tumour cell membrane. The result of this may be that the tumour will die or may not grow as fast, giving the immune system time to recognise and destroy the tumour. Secondly, a lower level of sugar in the blood will result in a lower level of insulin secretion from the pancreas being needed to deal with the sugar. The lower level of insulin secretion will mean less insulin is available to stimulate tumour growth.

As a result of the glucose drain that tumours exert, cancer patients become malnourished and tired. Many cancer patients experience a huge weight loss as the tumour demands more glucose, which may play a role in the condition known as cancer cachexia [43]. To counteract this weight loss, most hospitalised cancer patients are given a standard liquid intensive care diet. This diet is not specifically designed for cancer patients and can contain up to 30% glucose. This type of diet will actually feed the cancer more than the patient and the weight loss will continue. Non hospitalised cancer patients are often told by their doctors to eat a good healthy diet or to 'eat whatever you feel like.'

Cachexia is similar to the condition of partial starvation, as mentioned earlier, where a small amount of glucose switches off the protective starvation mechanism and causes muscle tissue to be broken down to yield glucose. This may prove a vital area for research, where ketosis could be switched on and tissue loss averted by giving cachexic patients a no carbohydrate, low protein and high fat diet. The aim must be to control blood sugar

45

levels within a narrow band. With further research the control of blood glucose levels is likely to become an important component of cancer treatment.

Insulin potentiation therapy: a new hope?

Using this principle of controlling blood glucose levels, an innovative treatment for cancer patients called insulin potentiation therapy has been devised [44]. This cancer treatment capitalises on the high glucose requirement of tumour cells and their excess of insulin receptors. The therapy involves the patient consuming a low carbohydrate, high protein and fat diet. This type of diet will keep blood insulin and blood sugar levels low. With insulin potentiation therapy, a measured amount of insulin is then injected into the blood stream, and this primes the cancer cells for sugar uptake. Instead of sugar, a chemotherapeutic agent (similar in structure to sugar) is added to the blood and the insulin stimulates its uptake by the tumour cells. This therapy effectively targets the tumour cells with the chemical agent and kills them. Only one tenth of the usual dose of chemotherapeutic agent is required, avoiding some of the unpleasant side effects of chemotherapy [45]. This is a relatively new cancer therapy, however, and is not yet widely practised, but results do look promising.

In the US, the consumption of sugar has increased from 126lb to in excess of 150lb per person per year in the past two decades. This trend has been clearly correlated with an increase in the incidence of diabetes [46]. The Western world is not alone, however. India has a diet rich in sugar and leads the world today with the largest number of diabetics in any country. In the 1970s, the prevalence of diabetes among urban Indians was reported to be 2.1% and this has now risen to 12.1% [47]. India now has approximately 20 million diagnosed diabetics. Moreover, there is an equally large pool of individuals with impaired glucose tolerance, many of whom will develop Type 2 diabetes mellitus in the future. However, this does not take into account undiagnosed individuals in the poorer regions of India where protein-poor, sugar-rich diets are consumed and doctors' fees unaffordable. As a result, the true figure may be much higher.

The sugar controversy: bad diets and big business

How much added sugar is it safe to eat in our daily diets? Answering this question is not as simple as it may first appear. The answer depends on who you want to believe, or who you trust. The sugar industry maintains that sugar can constitute 25% of the total daily calories of a healthy diet. Other organisations such as the WHO with no vested interest in sugar suggest that no more that 5% of daily calories should come from added sugar. We recommend eliminating sugar from the diet all together, especially if you have been diagnosed with cancer, heart disease or diabetes.

The World Health Organisation and sugar

The tobacco industry fought for two decades against the medical evidence that linked smoking to cancer, heart disease, emphysema and other illnesses. Millions of people died prematurely who may otherwise have given up smoking if the tobacco lobby and compliant scientists had not worked long and hard to confuse the customers. Tobacco companies are now under attack in the US as the courts award bigger and bigger settlements to its victims or their survivors, but the 20 years of confusion and misleading statements kept the huge profits rolling in for an extra 20 years, and still they roll in from the Third World.

In April 2003, the WHO put forward guidelines on their web site, to be published later, compiled from a panel of 30 world experts concerning nutrition and health [48]. In this preliminary report, experts proposed that no more than 10% of daily calories should be derived from added sugar. Recommendations made in the 150-page report include eating at least 400g of fruit and vegetables per day, and taking at least one hour of exercise per day.

The report, 'Diet, Nutrition and the Prevention of Chronic Diseases' was the result of a two year study by the United Nations Food and Agriculture Organisation (FAO) and the WHO. The report tackled the rapidly rising worldwide incidence of CVD, several forms of cancer, diabetes, obesity, osteoporosis and dental disease. These diseases, all of which are associated with diet, contributed 59% of the 56.5 million total reported deaths in the world in 2001, more than half of them in poor countries that can ill afford the costs of treating these diseases. This report did not detail the age ranges in the mortality figures.

In response to this report, the sugar industry in the US used all of the lessons learned by the tobacco industry before them. Initially, institutes were set up to throw doubt on the evidence. The International Life Sciences Institute, founded by Coca-Cola, Pepsico, General Foods, Proctor and Gamble, and Kraft, is now accredited to both the WHO and the FAO and produces evidence extolling the virtues of sugar and suggesting that apart from a minor role in dental caries, sugar does not cause any health problems. In addition to these proven strategies, just for good measure, the sugar industry threatened to bring the WHO to its knees by demanding that the US Congress end its funding unless the WHO scrapped their guidelines on healthy eating, which were published on Wednesday 23 April 2003. The threat was described in the popular press as tantamount to blackmail, and worse than any pressure exerted by the tobacco lobby in the past.

In a letter to Gro Harlem Brundtland, the WHO's director general, the Sugar Association said it would "exercise every avenue available to expose the dubious nature" of the WHO report on diet and nutrition, including challenging its $406m (£260m) funding from the US government.

The Sugar Association stated that "Tax dollars should not be used to support misguided, non-science-based reports which do not add to the health and wellbeing of Americans, much less the rest of the world. If necessary we will promote and encourage new laws which require future WHO funding to be provided only if the organisation accepts that all reports must be supported by the preponderance of scientific data available."

In a letter to Mr Tommy Thompson, the US Health Secretary at the time, the sugar lobby relied heavily on a recent report from the Institute of Medicine of the National Academies for its claim that a 25% sugar intake is acceptable. However, Harvey Fineberg, president of the Institute of Medicine, wrote to Mr Thompson to warn that the report was being misinterpreted. He said it did not make a recommendation on sugar intake. What the Institute of Medicine actually stated was that while the acceptable range of carbohydrates is 45 to 65% of total calories, the report suggested that no more than 25% of total calories should come from added sugar. However, the report did not lay down a specific sugar limit for achieving a healthy diet and lifestyle. The report also stated that individuals who consumed sugar at these levels were more likely to have a poor intake of important essential nutrients.

Speaking to the BBC on this subject, following the publication of the amended WHO report, Dr Pekka Puska, director of non-communicable disease at the WHO, suggested that big commercial interests "with major links" were trying to interfere. Pressure was "pretty high", he said, because the WHO has a very high status as a source on health information. "I don't think this is a very wise strategy by the industry, because the evidence is so strong and the public believes this message," said Dr Puska. "I think it is a bit short-sighted to deny the facts and it would be better to collaborate. Food is different from tobacco. We always have to eat, so our aim is just to change consumption from unhealthy to healthy."

The WHO is an independent body and relies on expert scientific evidence when making recommendations such as these. So for the WHO to put forward a recommendation of 10% of added sugar in a healthy diet was extremely significant. This recommendation was supported by a previous US government funded report in 2001–2002 (USDA Agricultural Fact book) which suggested an even lower healthy sugar level of 8%, for the average person on a 2,000-calorie daily diet.

What is behind the over consumption of sugar? One major factor is the success of the soft drink industry, and fast food restaurants, but the addictive nature of sugar is pivotal. This is exacerbated by the misconception that a fat-free food, no matter how high in sugar or calories, will not increase body fat. The Sugar Association plays a major role in influencing the perception of the public of the virtues of sugar in a healthy balanced diet. It also has a major influence with the food industry. The Association publishes a column in a scientific journal called the Journal of the American Dietetic Association (ADA). The ADA's 'position statement' on sugars was co-authored by an advisor to the Canadian sugar industry.

What can individuals do to reduce the amount of added sugars consumed each day? To begin with, the term 'added sugar' refers not only to the sugar added to tea, coffee, breakfast cereal and so on, but also to the sugar added by the manufacturers of many processed foods and drinks.

Most food labels now carry information relating to the recommended daily allowance (RDA) of many of the minor ingredients in that food, but with the exception of the major nutrients, protein, fat and sugar. RDAs for protein and fat are less important because variation of their content in foods and drinks is not a potential health hazard like sugar. If we accept the latest WHO recommendations of 27.5g of added sugar per day, then this should be the value for the RDA. A teaspoon of sugar is approximately 4g, whilst a can of cola will provide upto 40g of sugar.

Dietary advice

In general, all processed and quick energy foods such as sugar-rich foods should be avoided. These products can be very tempting, but the large number of serious and often life threatening diseases associated with their consumption suggests that they should be avoided at all costs. Most of us can already identify these products on the supermarket shelves if we stop to think about it. By law all these products must indicate the quantity of sugar within them. We must avoid being lured by attractive packaging and advertising gimmicks, and master our cravings for such foods.

Products that we need to cut down on and if possible cut out of our diet altogether include cakes, confectionery, canned fruit, chewing gum, chocolate, biscuits, fruit juices, ice cream, jams, jellies, pastries, pies, preserves, puddings, sherbets and soft drinks. We should also try to avoid products containing white, brown, powdered and icing sugars, corn syrup and glucose. All of these products have a high glycaemic index/load and are damaging to our health.

Artificial sweeteners

Side effects of aspartame

We should try not to use artificial sweeteners such as aspartame, saccharin and products containing them. Artificial sweeteners may seem an attractive alternative to sugar but they are associated with potentially serious health problems.

Aspartame is included in a huge variety of the foods we consume, not just in diet drinks. Relatively low doses of aspartame will significantly increase methanol levels in our blood [49]. Very low level exposure to methanol has been shown to cause headaches, dizziness, nausea, ear buzzing, gastrointestinal disturbances, weakness, vertigo, chills, memory lapses, numbness, shooting pains, behavioural disturbances, blurring of/ misty vision, conjunctivitis, vision loss, insomnia, depression, heart disease and pancreatic inflammation [50, 51].

Once in the body, methanol is converted into formaldehyde. In the days of the Prohibition in the US, methanol was responsible for thousands of cases of blindness, insanity and death due to the consumption of illicit wood alcohol. Continuous exposure to very low doses of formaldehyde has been shown to cause immune system and nervous system damage as well as headaches, general poor health and irreversible genetic damage [52–54]. It is perhaps significant that American Air Force pilots are not allowed to consume products containing aspartame. What are the alternatives then, if both sugar and artificial sweeteners pose an unacceptable health risk?

Xylitol, the healthy alternative

In our opinion there is only one product that has all the necessary qualities to replace sugar, and that is the sugar alcohol xylitol. It is a natural 5-carbon sugar alcohol found in some vegetables and fruit, such as cauliflowers and raspberries, and hardwood trees like birch. The human body makes about 15g per day during normal metabolism. It was discovered in the 1890s and then forgotten. It was then reassessed during World War 2 in Finland due to sugar shortages. Finnish chemists developed a process using birch bark and wood chips which contain hemicellulose, a polymer which they converted to xylitol. The process was very expensive and low post-war sugar prices prevented any serious exploitation. Currently it retails at about ten times the price of sugar in specialist health food shops. Despite its high price, it offers considerable health advantages as a sugar substitute.

- It looks and tastes very similar to sugar, without the unpleasant aftertaste of some other sweeteners.

- It is only slowly absorbed from the intestine. Only a third is absorbed and metabolised in the liver without the involvement of insulin. The remaining two thirds enters the large intestine where the resident bacteria convert it to short chain fatty acids, some of which are absorbed and metabolised by the body.

- It is therefore an ideal sugar substitute for diabetics, and has been used for some years in Japan and the US in specialist diabetic food products.

- It has a glycaemic index of only 7 (cf. glucose GI = 100) and supplies only 40% of the calories of an equivalent weight of sugar, making it an ideal component of low carbohydrate, calorie controlled diets.

- It cannot be fermented by yeasts and mouth bacteria that cause dental plaque and tooth decay. It also changes the pH of saliva from acidic to alkaline and chelates or binds calcium which may stimulate the re-calcification of tooth enamel.

- Consumption of xylitol has further beneficial health implications. It inhibits the growth in the nasal cavity of the beta-haemolytic streptococci and *Streptococcus pneumoniae*, which occur universally and are normally harmless, but can become a reservoir of infection in immune-compromised patients, often with fatal results.

- Dietary xylitol has been shown to protect children against otitis media.

- Critics of this compound as a dietary aid usually quote its effect on intestinal motility. Because it is able to reach the large intestine, overconsumption can lead to diarrhoea. However, as part of a specific calorie controlled diet, this problem should not arise and any small decrease in transit time should be considered a health benefit.

A number of other natural products can be used as sweeteners, such as raw unprocessed honey, Sucanat (dehydrated organic, raw sugar cane juice), palm sugar and barley malt or rice syrup. None are ideal as they all involve eating sugar. Fruit juice can be used for some baking (e.g. pineapple, apple). Since all sugars are potentially harmful, the best approach is to train one's palate to accept less sweet foods, with a lower sugar content.

Stevia, a safe non-sugar sweetener

This calorie-free sweetener from the South American plant *Stevia rebaudiana Bertoni* is 300 times as sweet as sugar and has been used for centuries as a natural sweetening agent. The pure steviol glycoside has been passed as safe in the US by the FDA and in Europe by the EFSA. It is an ideal replacement for sugar in diabetic diets.

White flour and white flour-containing food

It is important to avoid eating products made with white flour, such as white bread, dumplings, biscuits, buns, pizza, pasta and processed dry cereals. Other grains offer a greater range of flavour and nutrition than commercially processed, wheat-based products. Food products made from processed, finely milled white flour have a high glycaemic index/load and play a role in weight gain, diabetes and the development of heart disease. Whole grain flour (particularly from oats) has important cholesterol and TG lowering effects and may protect us from heart disease. This effect is reversed with refined white flour [55].

Healthy alternatives

It is advisable to include in the diet foods made from rye, quinoa, amaranth, oats, millet, brown and wild rice and brown pasta. The

North American Indians used buckwheat flour. If you must consume bread, eat 100% wholemeal bread. In recent studies, regular consumption of whole grain foods was associated with a reduction in the incidence of CVD and diabetes, reductions in mortality from certain cancers and an overall reduction in premature death [56]. The amount of refined carbohydrate in the bread you eat should be as low as possible. As an alternative, one could try whole grain crackers without polyunsaturated oils.

Grains, beans and pulses are good alternatives to flour-based products. It is advisable to avoid any grains or seeds that may have been contaminated with a yellow mould *Aspergillus flavis* which produces the deadly aflatoxin, known to cause a variety of cancers. While peas can be eaten raw, most beans need to be cooked to destroy potentially toxic lectins.

Dietary fibre and resistant starch: a re-evaluation

Research over the past 20 years has revealed some important differences in the roles of insoluble and soluble dietary fibres. Insoluble fibres such as cellulose and lignans play an important role in maintaining faecal bulk and intestinal health. Soluble fibres have a more important metabolic role. They are found in fruit, vegetables and cereals as pectins, gums, mucilages, hemicelluloses and resistant starch (RS). The metabolism of these soluble fibres is known to control blood glucose and cholesterol levels. Resistant starch is the most important member of the group, and its concentration in foods can be increased by cooking and processing. Like the other soluble dietary fibres, RS is fermented in the colon to provide long-term energy. It does not evoke an insulin response and is referred to as non-glycaemic carbohydrate. Resistant starch is a crucial dietary component for weight and blood glucose management and intestinal health.

Traditional diets rich in whole grains, vegetables and fibre have long been known to protect against obesity, diabetes Type 2, and several cancers. The major protective component in these diets, and often lacking in Western diets, is resistant starch. This is classed as the plant starch fraction that escapes digestion in the small intestine and passes into the colon. There it is slowly fermented by the resident bacteria to produce butyric acid which the main energy source for the cells of the colonic epithelium, the colonocytes. This production of butyrate protects against colon cancer, and helps to control blood glucose levels.

Dietary recommendations for resistant starch

Resistant starch consumption in the developed world is calculated at 3–7g/day. The WHO recommends a total dietary fibre (soluble + insoluble) intake of >25g/day, whereas the CSIRO in Australia recommend 20g/day of resistant starch for optimum bowel health. Some clinicians and nutritionists are now suggesting a daily intake of 25g for women and 40g for men for optimum health benefits since a high intake of resistant starch appears to have no unwanted side effects. Green bananas are a cheap and readily available source of resistant starch.

The unique dietary properties of resistant starch

- Gives some of the benefits of insoluble fibres as well as multiple benefits of soluble fibres.

- Improves the glycaemic response by increasing insulin sensitivity.

- Reduces obesity by stimulating fat oxidation.

- Reduces the inflammatory response.

- Helps to establish a healthy large bowel microflora.

- Reduces the risk of colon cancer by generating butyrate in the large bowel.

- Pure RS is gluten free and can replace flour in wheat-free and coeliac diets.

- Lowers the calorie content of foods by 50% when replacing refined flour or sugars.

- The physical properties of RS allow it to be incorporated into normal foods like bread, pastries, cakes, biscuits and drinks without causing consumer rejection.

- Reduces hunger pangs for two to three hours in the short term and 20–24 hours in the longer term.

- Helps to maintain bowel regularity by increasing microbial activity in the large intestine, to cause a mild laxative effect.

The facts listed above reveal how important resistant starch is as a crucial component of a healthy diet.

4 Dietary protein

Proteins are large molecules consisting of chains of amino acids joined together by peptide bonds. Of the 20 different amino acids found in proteins, eight are essential and must be obtained from the diet. The remaining 12 are termed non-essential and can be made in the body. Proteins are essential for cell structure and function and play a role in virtually all biological processes. A healthy human diet must contain a minimum of 10–20% of the total dietary calories as protein. They are digested in the stomach and intestine to release amino acids which are absorbed in the small intestine, and largely incorporated into body proteins which are in a constant state of turnover. Animal and fish proteins are the best sources of essential amino acids. Vegetarians must consume a variety of plant proteins to ensure an adequate supply of essential amino acids. Proteins can be broken down to release energy via glucose during starvation or when a high protein, low carbohydrate diet is consumed.

Introduction

Proteins are the main component molecules of life. The body uses proteins for growth and to build and repair bone, muscles, connective tissue, skin, internal organs and blood. Hormones, antibodies and the enzymes that regulate the body's chemical reactions are all made of protein.

59

All proteins are made up of different combinations of just 20 simple compounds called amino acids. The proteins we eat are broken down into peptides in the stomach by the enzyme pepsin, and into amino acids by enzymes secreted from the pancreas. These amino acids are then taken up by the intestines and metabolised by the liver. All amino acids can then be used as building blocks for new proteins involved in metabolism, growth or tissue repair. A sub-group called the glucogenic (glucose forming) amino acids can be converted into glucose for maintaining blood sugar in the body during periods of starvation or low carbohydrate consumption.

Dietary protein requirements

Dietary proteins contain two forms of amino acid, eight essential and 12 non-essential. The body makes non-essential amino acids but the eight essential amino acids must be obtained from the diet, usually from a combination of animal and plant proteins. In order to obtain an adequate supply of these essential amino acids, only 10 to 20% of the daily calorific intake needs to be in the form of protein [48].

Our recomendation for phyisically active adults is to consume 15% of your calories as protein, which equates to 93g a day for a 70kg (154lb) male. This is slighty less than the daily average consumed in America. Over consumption may be associated with health problems, particularly for inactive individuals who will not need much protein for muscle repair and growth. Such individuals should reduce their protein consumption towards the RDA for sedentary adults which is 56g/day (again for a 70kg male).

Protein content of foods

Since fresh foods are not sold with detailed contents labels, it is useful to get a general idea of the composition of basic foods. An excellent source of this kind of data is '*The Healthy Diet Calorie Counter*' by Kirsten Hartvig. Some representative examples of the proportion of protein to be found in a variety of foods are shown in Table 2 (pg 62). The protein content of many common foods is shown as g per portion, which can readily be converted to g per 100g for ease of comparison.

Meat, fish, eggs and cheese are the most concentrated source of quality animal protein, with legumes (peas, beans and lentils), nuts and seeds being the plant protein-rich alternatives. Nuts and grain contain more than 10% of their calories as protein, as do fruit and vegetables, but all foods contain varying amounts of water which will lower the actual concentration of protein in the food. For example, to obtain 56g of protein from one food alone it would be necessary to consume either 14kg of apples, 7kg of lettuce, 240g of roast beef, 156g of Parmesan cheese, or 15 slices (600g) of wholemeal bread (see table 2, pg 62).

Based on the daily protein requirement, Table 2 can be used to design a healthy, balanced range of protein sources. Eating enough protein each day for a healthy existence almost certainly provides enough calories because in food, protein is typically associated with carbohydrate and fat. Sugar-rich, low protein junk food diets may not supply adequate protein. We must also remember that the RDA guidelines have to be flexible to take account of the increased protein requirements of women who are pregnant or breastfeeding, and for those who undertake high intensity exercise.

61

Table 2 **Proportions of protein in some common foods**

Food	Portion size (g)	Protein (g)
Almonds	50	10.6
Apple	100	0.4
Baked beans	130	6.2
Banana	100	1.2
Bran flakes	50	7.6
Broccoli	100	4.2
Cheeses (average)	40	9.0
Chicken	120	27.1
Chips	180	6.1
Corn flakes	50	4.0
Egg	50	6.3
Fish (average)	120	20.0
Lentils (cooked)	100	8.8
Lettuce	80	0.7
Melon	180	1.1
Milk	200 ml	6.8
Nut roast	130	20.0
Parmesan cheese	40	14.5
Peanuts	50	12.8
Pear	170	0.5
Pizza (cheese & tomato)	300	27.3
Quorn	100	11.8
Roast beef	120	28.1
Watercress	80	2.4
Wholemeal bread (one slice)	40	3.7
Yoghurt (average)	150	8.0

When it comes to readily available information concerning health and nutrition, the role of proteins in a healthy diet has been largely overshadowed by interest in the roles of fat, carbohydrates and vitamins. While the RDA for protein is well established, the upper dietary limit is less clear. Also, relatively little is known of the functions of different proteins in nutrition and health. As a result, much of the information we have concerning high protein diets is historical or anecdotal. Arctic explorers have survived for many months on a diet of seal meat and blubber without apparent ill effects. Labourers building the Great Western Railway in the US are said to have subsisted mainly on a pemmican diet (dried buffalo meat and fat). Some scientific studies have been carried out on high fat/protein diets based on the Inuit and Masai cultures, and the many millions of people with experience of low-glycaemic, Atkins-type diets could provide a useful source of data in the future.

Protein and dietary misconceptions

Critics of high fat/protein/low carbohydrate diets often quote a flawed study in 1905 [57], which proposed that 50% of dietary protein was converted to sugar. This was proposed to raise blood sugar and insulin levels as would a carbohydrate diet. Later research [58–60] demonstrated that a high protein diet did not cause a significant rise in the blood glucose levels of normal or diabetic subjects. In addition, the perceived link between high protein diets and kidney stones is not supported, but protein restricted diets help patients with kidney disease [61]. However, eating a high protein diet with adequate fat does not cause kidney problems because the dietary fat-soluble vitamins and saturated fatty acids associated with animal proteins or plant proteins are vital for properly functioning kidneys [62].

63

High or low protein diets

Insufficient dietary protein can be unhealthy and even fatal [63]. Lack of protein can cause retardation of growth, loss of muscle, decreased immunity [64], weakening of the heart [65] and the respiratory system [66], mental retardation and death. These symptoms are seen in severely malnourished children as infantile marasmus and are largely irreversible. Too little protein is clearly a problem but can we get too much protein in our diet? Some research has suggested that eating a high protein diet may result in too much calcium being excreted in the urine. During protein digestion there is a release of acids into the blood. This acidity is largely neutralised by calcium. On average, 1mg of calcium may be lost in urine for every 1g rise in protein consumed in the diet [67]. This loss of calcium may affect bone strength.

Can we eat too much protein?

Eating a high protein diet for a few weeks will not have much effect on bone strength. However, in the long term, a high protein diet without calcium supplementation may weaken bones, as was suggested by the results of the Nurses' Health Study. In this study, women who ate more than 95g of protein a day were 20% more likely to have broken a wrist over a 12 year period compared to those who consumed an average amount of protein (less than 68g a day), but calcium intake and urinary loss were not measured [68]. However, a recent scientific study has suggested that increasing dietary protein does not affect the amount of calcium excreted in the urine, but has been associated with higher circulating levels of a bone growth factor in the blood. This suggests that a high protein diet would enhance bone strength [69], but only in the presence of adequate dietary calcium to compensate for the increased calcium loss associated with the breakdown of protein for energy.

The role of protein in bone strength appears complex and is not fully understood, although it probably depends on age, health, exercise and the presence of other nutrients in the diet. What is apparent is that a balanced diet with ample fruit and vegetables and adequate protein seems important for bone mineral density [70]. Recent research supports this, with particular reference to the consumption of dark green vegetables such as broccoli, kale, cabbage and spinach. In addition to valuable antioxidants, these vegetables are a rich source of vitamin K_1 which plays a crucial role in bone formation and the prevention of osteoporosis and calcification (hardening) of the arteries. Surveys show that subjects with low blood levels of vitamins K_1 or K_2 are more prone to limb fractures and osteoarthritis.

Myth of milk as a good source of protein and calcium

As part of a healthy diet, milk has long been thought of as an excellent source of both protein and minerals and is associated with dietary calcium and strong bones. Milk is undoubtedly a good source of protein. However, it is not a good source of calcium for bone strength. In a 12-year Harvard study of 78,000 women, it was found that those who drank milk three times a day actually broke more bones than women who rarely drank milk. Similarly, a study of elderly Australian men and women showed that higher dairy product consumption was associated with increased bone fracture risk. Furthermore, those with the highest dairy product consumption had approximately double the risk of hip fracture compared to those with the lowest consumption [71]. This may be partly as a result of the high level of phosphate in

65

milk. Phosphate in cow's milk may bind with calcium in the digestive tract and sharply reduces its absorption. A more controversial reason may be that the protein in milk, as with other high protein foods, leads to a build-up of acid in our blood. Calcium is leached from bones to neutralise this acid. So milk may actually be no good for our bones at all.

Which proteins are the healthiest to consume?

Proteins can come from a variety of different sources. Some of the protein will contain all the amino acids needed to make new proteins. This kind of protein is called complete protein. Animal proteins are usually complete. Proteins that lack essential amino acids are termed incomplete proteins. These usually come from fruits, vegetables, grains, and nuts. The consumption of a combination of different plant proteins, termed complementation, can supply the complete range of amino acids needed by the body, so with planning, vegetarians can get all the protein they need for a healthy lifestyle from plant material.

Protein complementation for vegetarians

The three essential amino acids which are most commonly lacking in plant foods are lysine (Lys), tryptophan (Trp) and methionine (Met). Table 3 lists common plant foods and their relative composition of the three essential amino acids most lacking in vegetarian diets. These three amino acids can be obtained by varying the type of plant food consumed. Thus, combining corn and beans can use the excess lysine in beans to offset the shortage of lysine in corn. This is the basis of the staple Central American diet, with rice and beans being important in many Asian diets. In fact, beans form the most important source of lysine to complement all the carbohydrate-rich foods in Table 3, and are a crucial component of vegan and vegetarian diets.

In terms of healthy eating, we recommend a diet with a higher proportion of plant proteins than animal proteins. One reason for this is that cooking certain meats at high temperatures results in the formation of toxic substances that are known to have a negative effect on health. Examples of these substances are heterocyclic aromatic amines and polycyclic aromatic hydrocarbons, which are formed when meats such as beef, lamb, pork, fowl and fish are cooked at high temperatures [72]. These high temperatures are most often achieved by roasting, grilling or barbecuing meat. These toxic substances, some of which may be cancer causing agents [73], are formed when amino acids and creatine (found in muscles) react together at high temperature. The same will apply to the cooking of plant material under excessive heat, but this tends not to occur when cooking plant products as they are usually steamed or boiled.

Table 3 **Essential amino acids in basic foods**

	Essential amino acids [a]		
Protein source	**Lys**	**Trp**	**Met**
Corn (maize)	−	−	+
Wheat	−	+	−
Rice	−	+	+
Potato	+	+	−
Beans	++	−	+

[a] − deficiency, + adequate

Weight control

In short-term studies, a diet that involves eating less carbohydrate and more protein and fat is more effective for losing weight or keeping weight steady than a high carbohydrate, low protein, low fat diet [74]. Eating foods high in protein such as beef, chicken, fish or beans reduces hunger pangs because the food is released more slowly from the stomach to the intestine. This may help to reduce and delay hunger and can lead to eating fewer calories.

Eating protein maintains the steady state blood glucose concentration at approximately 100mg/ml without the peaks and troughs associated with sugar consumption. Insulin secretion after a protein meal is extremely low when compared to the amount secreted after a carbohydrate-rich meal. Eating protein-rich, low carbohydrate meals avoids the rapid increases and drops in blood sugar that can trigger the feeling of hunger. This type of diet can also help diabetics to control blood sugar levels and insulin requirements. Highs and lows in blood sugar are common in people who eat quick energy foods such as refined carbohydrates, and as a result they experience hunger sooner after a meal.

At present, very few studies have been performed concerning the long-term effects of a high-protein/fat diet on weight control, although the number of studies is increasing rapidly and we will be in a better position in the near future to evaluate the health aspects of such diets.

Protein and chronic disease

Dietary protein may play a significant role in protection from a number of chronic diseases such as obesity, heart disease, diabetes and cancer.

Heart disease

One large prospective study performed in 1999 investigated the association between dietary protein and heart disease. In this study [75], women who ate the most protein (approximately 110g per day) were 25% less likely to have had a heart attack and/or die of heart disease than the women who ate the least protein (about 68g per day) over a 14-year period. The source of the protein, animal or vegetable or whether it was part of a fat controlled diet did not seem to be important. These results suggested that eating a high protein diet does not harm the heart. Eating more protein while cutting back on easily digested carbohydrates may actually benefit the heart, by lowering insulin levels which controls fat production.

More recently in 2003 a study has suggested that an increased intake of protein, particularly plant protein, may lower blood pressure and reduce the risk of CVD [76]. Many reports have suggested that soy food products can help reduce the risk of heart disease [77–79].

In 1995, an analysis of 38 controlled clinical trials indicated that eating approximately 50g of soy protein a day in place of animal protein played a role in reducing serum TGs by 10.5%. The reduction in serum TG is now thought to be far more important than the effect on serum cholesterol [80]. Such reductions could potentially mean a reduction in the risk of developing heart disease in a high risk population. So, from this we can say that eating a high protein diet does not harm the heart. A note of caution should be introduced here with respect to diets rich in soy products causing acquired mineral deficiency.

Diabetes

Proteins found in cow's milk may play a role in the development of Type 1 diabetes (insulin dependent diabetes or juvenile diabetes). This is one reason why cow's milk is not universally recommended for infants [81]. Other studies have disputed these findings and suggested that the protein in milk is not responsible for development of Type 1 diabetes. Later in life the amount of protein in the diet does not seem to adversely affect the development of Type 2 diabetes (adult onset), although research in this area is ongoing.

Cancer

There is no conclusive evidence that eating too little or too much protein will increase cancer risk. However, soy-based foods including soy protein have been suggested to play a role in the prevention of breast and prostate cancer [82]. These claims made for soy products may be thanks to the high concentrations of isoflavones, which are forms of plant oestrogen or phytoestrogen. For this reason it has been suggested that soy products are protective against breast cancer.

The phytoestrogens in soy protein foods may act to block the binding of oestrogens to receptors on the surface of tumour cells, thus blocking oestrogen dependent tumour growth. If this occurs in breast tissue, then eating soy may play a role in reducing the risk of breast cancer. However, up to now scientific studies have not provided clear evidence of this effect. Some studies have shown a benefit and others show no association between soy consumption and breast cancer [83]. Some reports suggest that concentrated supplements of soy protein may actually stimulate the growth of breast cancer cells [84]. It has also been suggested that soy may be involved in the development of pancreatic cancer [85] and may play a role in the development of other forms of cancer [86], the depression of thyroid function [87], and interfere with mineral and vitamin uptake from food, potentially leading to stunted growth.

Soybeans are high in a substance called phytic acid. This substance can block the intestinal uptake of essential minerals such as calcium, magnesium, copper, iron and especially zinc. Many scientists agree that diets high in phytates derived from soy have contributed to widespread mineral deficiencies in Third World countries, even in areas where minerals are not in short supply. If soy causes mineral deficiencies, the question that arises is how have the Japanese consumed soy for generations with no apparent damaging health effects. Traditionally, the Japanese eat a small amount of tofu or miso as part of a mineral rich fish broth, followed by a serving of meat or fish. It is important to know that miso and other traditional Japanese foods such as natto are soya bean products which have been fermented with *Bacillus subtilis* strains which lower the phytic acid and isoflavone content of these foods. It seems that the negative qualities of unfermented soy are more than compensated for by other nutritious components in the Japanese diet. However, if vegetarians consume tofu and bean curd as a total substitute for meat, they will be at risk of severe mineral deficiencies.

Animal protein will invariably be associated with animal fat consumption. It is extremely difficult to separate the two to any great extent. A diet that is high in animal protein and low in carbohydrate will usually be a diet rich in fat, unless lean meat such as chicken and non-oily fish are selected. The consequences of a fat-rich diet are discussed in the next chapter.

Dietary advice

Unhealthy types of meat

If possible, one should try to avoid eating chicken raised in battery conditions, as much for health reasons as for moral and ethical reasons. Battery chickens tend to be exposed to more chemicals and diseases than free range chickens.

The consumption of excessive amounts of smoked meats or luncheon meats, sausage, hot dogs, salami, bologna and pastrami should be avoided. Many of these meats contain significant levels of nitrate or nitrite. Consuming these compounds in the diet has been shown to induce stomach and colorectal cancer [88]. If possible, one should avoid eating too much of any meats that are processed, salted or preserved, unless consumed with adequate amounts of antioxidant-rich salads, and water to counteract the salt.

Healthy alternatives

The consumer should choose organic beef, free-range chicken and poultry. Game birds and animals are low in saturated fat and contaminating chemicals and hormones. The method of preparation of meat is important. As far as possible, we would recommend baking or poaching meat and avoiding excessive broiling/grilling and frying. Although it is extremely tempting, especially in the summer, one should avoid consuming too much barbecued meat. These meats contain carcinogens formed from the oxidation of fat and protein [89]. If you must barbecue meat, make sure you eat plenty of fresh salad vegetables and fruit to counteract the potential damaging effects of the burned meat. It is worth mentioning that the compounds responsible for lung cancer found in cigarette smoke are very similar to those produced on the surface of a barbecued joint (polycyclic aromatic hydrocarbons (PAHs), such as benzopyrene).

Seafood is an excellent source of nutrition but must be fresh. Oily fish is a good source of omega-3 fatty acids and micronutrients. A healthy diet should contain at least one meal of fish per week. It is advisable to avoid eating too much smoked, salted, fried or breaded fish. As for shellfish, shrimp, clams, scallops and lobster, be careful of their origin. These fish are scavengers or filter feeders and can often retain relatively high levels of contaminants and pollutants in their bodies. Some fish such as tuna contain relatively high levels of mercury and should not be eaten more than once a week. This having been said, the benefits of consuming seafood far outweigh the risks.

The heavy metal story may have been overplayed, and it should be remembered that many more people become ill through the microbial spoilage of seafood and fresh foods in general. Bacteria present as faecal contaminants in some prepared fresh foods, such as *E. coli*, *Clostridia*, *Salmonella* and *Campylobacter*, have caused serious food poisoning outbreaks often with fatal consequences. Some of these bacteria can survive and even grow slowly in chilled food products, which are becoming increasingly popular as 'healthy' food options. It has been calculated that tens of thousands of people in the UK and hundreds of thousands in the US become ill through bacterial food poisoning. This represents only those who were ill enough to notify a doctor.

You can eat two eggs three to four times a week. Make sure that they are soft boiled, poached, lightly scrambled, or fried, and try to avoid hard-boiled eggs. Contrary to what you may have previously understood, eggs do not raise serum cholesterol or blood pressure [90, 91].

Some vegetarians tend to get their protein from processed food sources such as vegetarian sausages, burgers and other textured protein products made from Quorn and soy protein. These foods invariably contain partially hydrogenated fat and should be avoided. Vegetarians should limit their intake of soy protein for reasons indicated earlier in this chapter.

Egg and cheese products contain high quality protein and fat and can be supplemented with protein from legumes. True vegans have more of a problem obtaining a diet balanced in protein and need to eat a wide variety of plant products. Some vegetarians supplement their diets with oily fish; this is an excellent idea as the fish provide protein and essential omega-3 polyunsaturated fatty acids.

Dairy products

Commercial ice cream and dessert toppings such as cream substitutes should be avoided, and one should try to reduce milk consumption. A study of elderly Australian men and women showed that higher dairy product consumption was associated with increased fracture risk. Further, those with the highest dairy product consumption had approximately double the risk of hip fracture compared to those with the lowest consumption [71].

Cows milk contains a high level of soluble phosphate which can react with calcium salts under the alkaline conditions of the intestine to form insoluble calcium phosphate salts which cannot be absorbed. One should also avoid consuming powdered milk and sweetened yogurts (see section on artificial sweeteners in Chapter 3).

We are the only species that drinks the milk of another animal. Moreover, milk is produced to maximise the growth and development of the immature animals and contains growth factors that may play a role in the development of human cancers. Many health-conscious people accept skimmed milk as a healthy low fat alternative to full cream milk. It should be noted that reduced fat milk may contain added powdered milk to 'improve' palatability. The production of milk powder causes oxidation of cholesterol and recent research has indicated that it is oxidised cholesterol that is a risk factor in heart disease [92]. This is the same product that Kritchevsky fed to rabbits to induce atherosclerosis and to support his theory about the role of cholesterol in heart disease.

A Final warning:
Very high protein diets can be lethal. Chapter 2 describes how early Arctic explorers were well aware of the dangers of consuming too much protein in the absence of fat and carbohydrate. Several suffered protein poisoning and some died [11, 14]. This has particular relevance to modern dieting when protein is perceived as being healthy and fat as unhealthy. The latest advice for any diet is to limit protein intake to 1gm per Kg body weight per day.

5   Dietary fats: a question of balance?

Eating fat is essential and eating the right fats in the right proportions can optimise our health. Here we dispel the myth that very low fat diets are good for you and good for slimming, and present substantial evidence to the contrary. We look at which fats are essential and which to avoid, and how saturated, monounsaturated and polyunsaturated fats all contribute to a healthy diet. The beneficial properties of omega-3 fats are explained. We describe why chemically hydrogenated fats, containing industrial trans fats, and high concentrations of fats containing linoleate (omega-6) are very bad for our health. Fat chemistry is complex and the non-scientific reader is advised to skim the chemistry and concentrate on the molecules' properties and effects.

Introduction

The role of dietary fat is one of the most studied areas of nutrition and health. Dietary fat is essential for nutrition, but there is a distinct lack of scientific evidence concerning the role of natural fats in the development of chronic disease.

Definitions

Lipids

This is the generic term which encompasses all fats and sterols including cholesterol. The terms fat and fatty acid are often confused: fatty acids are a component of fat. Fat refers to the dietary source and to the storage material in fatty tissues. It is formed from glycerol which is derived from glucose, and is combined with fatty acids of varying chain length. The chemical name of fat is triglyceride or triacylglycerol (TG).

Fat is essential for life and normal body function. Fatty or adipose tissue serves to protect internal organs, and fatty acids are vital in cell membranes. Fat in adipose tissue insulates and helps to maintain body temperature, as well as acting as a crucial store of calories when food is scarce or absent. In addition, it functions as a storage depot for the oil-soluble vitamins and pigments. Blood lipids are involved in the transport of fat-soluble vitamins into and around the body. The brain is 60% fat, which serves to insulate nerve fibres.

Saturated fatty acids

In animals, the saturated fatty acid (SFA) series ranges from acetate, which has a two carbon side chain, and is not found in fat, to stearate, with 18 carbon atoms and which is a common constituent of human and animal fats. SFAs have straight side chains. They are completely saturated with hydrogen atoms and confer rigidity to cell membranes.

Medium chain fatty acids

Fats containing SFAs with six to 12 carbon atoms in their side chains are called medium chain fatty acids (MCFAs) and have some beneficial properties. They are readily digested and absorbed without the need for bile secretion, are oxidised as fuel and are not deposited in body fat. They can be used as slimming aids, in diets for athletes and in special diets for patients following liver operations or with impaired liver function.

Medium chain fatty acids are particularly well assimilated by new-born infants. The main source of these fats is coconut oil.

Unsaturated fatty acids

These fatty acids are formed from their saturated precursors by enzymes called desaturases, which remove hydrogen atoms from the side chains to form double bonds. The double bonds cause kinks to form in the side chains so that the molecules cannot stack closely together. As a consequence, unsaturated fats are generally liquids, and counteract the effects of SFAs to control the fluidity of cell membranes. All the saturated and the monounsaturated fats required in human metabolism can be made in the body and are therefore referred to as non-essential fatty acids. Fatty acids with more than one double bond are referred to as polyunsaturated fatty acids (PUFAs). Certain PUFAs cannot be made in the body and must be supplied in the diet, and are referred to as essential fatty acids. Table 4 lists the commonly available essential (E) and non-essential (NE) fatty acids (FAs).

Industrial trans fatty acids

These unnatural compounds are produced when TGs from vegetable oils and fats are chemically treated in a process known as partial hydrogenation in order to modify their properties for cooking, and to reduce their tendency to oxidise and become rancid. Trans fats are more specifically described as TGs containing partially hydrogenated fatty acids (trans fatty acids). To distinguish between the healthy trans fats found in cow's milk and the artificial, toxic trans fats formed by the above processes, we will refer to the latter as 'industrial trans fats' or ITFs.

Starting materials for the synthesis of omega-3 and 6 fatty acids

Linoleic acid is the parent acid for the omega-6 series of PUFAs, whereas α-linolenic acid is the precursor for the omega-3 series of PUFAs. These fatty acids are found in plants and contain only 18 carbon atoms in the side chain. They are often referred to as short chain PUFAs. In the absence of these essential fatty acids, the other PUFAs shown in Table 4 must be supplied in the diet. Saturated and unsaturated fats can be interconverted in the body with no toxic side effects; however, the chemical conversion of polyunsaturated fats by hydrogenation results in the formation of unnatural ITFs which have toxic side effects when present in the diet. The food industry has used this hydrogenation process for at least 100 years to modify the physical properties of vegetable oils for baking, cooking and better storage properties.

Omega-3 and omega-6 essential fatty acids

Of the three omega-6 fatty acids shown in Table 4, linoleate is by far the most commonly found PUFA in the vegetable, seed and nut oils which have now largely replaced the animal fats traditionally used in cooking. This dietary change has resulted in a massive imbalance in the ratio of omega-3 to omega-6 fatty acids in the diet.

Omega-3 and omega-6 fats are essential to health, and are vital for normal growth and development, but excessive consumption of omega-6 fats can have damaging side effects through stimulating the process of inflammation. Both the total amount and the even ratio between these fats are important, as they compete for conversion in the body to powerful hormone-like substances called prostaglandins that govern nearly every biological function.

Table 4 **Sources of fatty acids**

Type of fatty acid	Source
Saturated (NE)	
Acetic	Vinegar
Butyric	Butter
Palmitic	Tropical fats: coconut, palm and palm kernel
Stearic	Beef, mutton, pork, butter and cocoa butter
Monounsaturated (NE)	
Oleic (omega-9)	Large amounts in olives, avocado, peanuts, sesame, almonds, rapeseed/ canola, land animal fat and butter
Polyunsaturated (E)	
Omega-6 series	
Linoleic	Maize, safflower, hemp, sunflower, soy bean, walnut, pumpkin, cotton and flax seeds
γ-Linolenic	Borage, evening primrose and blackcurrant seed oils
Arachidonic	Meat and other animal products
Omega-3 series	
α-Linolenic	Flax and hemp seeds, soy beans and dark green leaves
Eicosapentaenoic (EPA)	Cold water fish, salmon, trout, mackerel and sardines
Docosahexaenoic (DHA)	Cold water fish, salmon, trout, mackerel and sardines

There are 'friendly' prostaglandins that enhance health, made from omega-3 oils, and proinflammatory prostaglandins that can be bad for the health, made from omega-6 oils to stimulate the immune system in response to pathogens. Excessive consumption of omega-6 fats leads to the over-production of arachidonic acid, the immediate precursor of the proinflammatory prostaglandins. In addition, omega-6 fats predominate in grains fed to livestock, leading to higher omega-6:omega-3 ratios in the fat of grain-fed cattle and chickens when compared to the ratios found in those fed solely on grass.

Omega-3 oils were initially discovered by Drs Burr and Burr in the 1930s, during a study of the Inuit, who consumed high levels of fish oil, which is rich in omega-3 fatty acids. The results of their studies indicated an extremely low incidence of heart disease and cancer amongst the traditional Inuit. Since then, numerous studies have suggested that omega-3 oil is good for our health. The higher fish intakes of the Japanese population relative to those of North America and many parts of Europe have been associated with their considerably lower rates of acute blocking of arteries, and other forms of heart disease, despite there being only moderately lower blood cholesterol levels in the Japanese population [93, 94]. Indeed, studies have suggested that diets that are rich in omega-3 fatty acids are inversely correlated with CHD disease in men [95].

Industrial production of trans fats

A large industry has developed to extract and process many oils from plant materials. While these processes can lead to oxidation and denaturation of many of the essential components, when properly controlled, they play a crucial role in preventing oxidation and hydrolysis. This is achieved by degumming which removes phospholipids and metals. However, refining invariably leads to the loss of crucial antioxidants like the tocopherols (E vitamins) and carotenoids (red and yellow oil-soluble plant pigments) which protect the polyunsaturated fats from oxidation. Some of these oils, particularly the commonly used edible oils from soy bean, maize, sunflower and rapeseed (canola), are partially hydrogenated to make solid fats for margarines and shortenings or to prevent rancidity when used as cooking oils. The most unstable omega-3 containing polyunsaturated fats are rapidly converted to trans fats in this process and the ratio of omega-3 to omega-6 fats is reduced leading to a less healthy product. There are three types of hydrogenation leading either to oils, margarines or hard cooking fats.

Industrial trans fats are poison fats

For the past 50 years at least, propaganda from the food industry has spread the notion that saturated fats (particularly animal fats such as butter and lard) are bad for health, and that margarine and vegetable oils are a healthier alternative. Much recent research contradicts this assertion. Recently, it has been suggested that vegetable fats play a role in the development of diabetes Type 2 in women. The risk arose due to ITF consumption. Margarine was the major dietary source of ITFs.

A study which began in 1980 with results published recently involved a review of medical and dietary data from over 84,000 healthy women. Results suggested that intake of total fat, saturated fat and monounsaturated fat did not influence diabetes risk [96]. However, the study also suggested that a 2% increase in calories from ITFs raised the risk of development of diabetes Type 2 in these women by 39% and a 5% increase in calories from polyunsaturated fat lowered the risk by 37%. ITF has often been called 'phantom fat' because food companies did not have to list the amount of ITF on food labels (this has changed in the

US and Denmark and changed in the UK in 2007). Canada led the way with ITF labelling from January, 2003.

So where does this fat come from? It would be hard to find beef fat or other solid animal fats in today's margarines and cooking oils. Soybean oil is the most common base; manufacturers also use sunflower, corn, palm, safflower, cottonseed, peanut and canola oils. They can do so only because about a century ago French and German chemists worked out how to convert liquid vegetable oils into a semi-solid product through hydrogenation. They heated the oil in the presence of a metal catalyst and pressurised hydrogen gas, causing hydrogen atoms to add randomly to the liquid fat. Complete hydrogenation saturates all double bonds, while partial hydrogenation saturates some. Over the past century, margarine makers have favoured partially hydrogenated oils, which remain soft enough for spreading and can then be made into shortening and margarine, and will have a longer shelf life. With the proliferation of processed foods, a long list of products now contain ITF. Even the vegetable oils labelled high in polyunsaturated fats, often chosen as a healthy dietary option, have been partially hydrogenated to prevent them going rancid and therefore contain ITF.

In the past there has been much publicity concerning the dangers of butter in the diet and suggesting that margarine is a much healthier option. This is totally untrue, and these statements were made without adequate evidence. ITFs are unique in that they affect our blood lipids (fats) in almost every possible way that is harmful to our health. We have just mentioned a suggested role in the development of Type 2 diabetes. ITFs also raise the proportion of 'bad' cholesterol (LDL) [97, 98] in the blood. Further, a study performed in 1994 showed that almost three quarters of the fat found clogging arteries is trans fat rather than cholesterol and comes from artificially hydrogenated ITF containing vegetable oils and cooking oils, not animal fats [99].

University of Maryland researchers led by Dr Mary Enig confirmed estimates that the average American consumed at least 12g of ITF per day. In addition, these workers suggested that those who consciously avoided animal fats typically consumed far more than 12g of trans fat per day. As far back as 1981 a study involving feeding trials showed that swine that were fed trans fatty acids developed a higher incidence of heart disease than those fed saturated fats, especially when ITFs were combined with added linoleate-rich polyunsaturates [100].

A study of Swedish women showed no correlation between saturated fat consumption and increased risk for breast cancer. However, the study did show a strong link between vegetable oil intake (containing ITFs) and higher breast cancer rates [101, 102]. More recent evidence has suggested that the apparent link between total fat intake and breast cancer was beginning to fade [103]. ITFs, as opposed to saturated fats, have also been shown to be causative factors in atherosclerosis, cancer and other diseases [104]. Changes in the consumption of these fats can be seen in Figure 6. This shows the potential dilemma of replacing animal fats with partially hydrogenated vegetable oils. As far back as 1978, Enig and co-workers had shown, through analysis of published results, a strong *positive* correlation with total fat (animal plus vegetable) but a strong *negative* correlation or no correlation with animal fat alone, to total cancer deaths, breast and colon cancer mortality and breast and colon cancer incidence. In other words, the use of vegetable oils seemed to predispose to heart disease and cancer and the use of animal fats seemed to protect [105].

85

When did the switch to partially hydrogenated vegetable oils occur? Margarine did have a major advantage in that it is cheaper to produce than butter, as a result of production from whale and vegetable oils use increased dramatically during the first half of the 20th century. At this time, legislation concerned with regulation of food content and labelling of products was not as stringent as it is today. To counteract growing public concern in the US, the Food, Drug and Cosmetic Act was passed in 1938, partly in response to consumer concerns about the adulteration of ordinary foodstuffs.

Dietary changes arising from warnings of the links between margarine consumption and increased heart disease should have led to a reduction in ITF consumption. However, any benefits were offset by changes in the type of fat used by the fast food industry; that is, the small decline in margarine consumption was overwhelmed by massive increases in the use of partially hydrogenated edible oil and baking fat consumption (see Figure 6). This also coincides with an increase in carbohydrate consumption and an increased rate of obesity incidence (see Figures 4 and 5 respectively).

The early 1980s were a time of rapid change in the food processing industry and an increase in the consumption of processed and fast foods. This increased use of hydrogenated fat was to be aided by the US Centre for Science in the Public Interest, which campaigned against the use of beef dripping for frying potatoes. As a result, most fast food concerns switched to partially hydrogenated soybean oil for frying foods; some deep frying oils contained almost 50% ITF.

Partially hydrogenated oils in general have enjoyed a hugely profitable history in the past 100 years. Significant factors leading to this success include a relatively cheap production and an aggressive marketing strategy. The marketing of margarine is largely based around its supposed health promoting properties. Margarine is marketed as a product low in cholesterol and rich in polyunsaturates which as a result will promote heart health when used in place of butter. Partially hydrogenated fats, until quite recently, were the principal fat in many prepared foods.

Until the food labelling law changes took effect, the only way to know whether a food contained ITF was to read the list of ingredients. If you see the words 'partially hydrogenated' in front of any vegetable oil, look for another brand that does not include these fats. In many instances this may prove difficult, as packaging for many food products does not at present contain any reference to content of hydrogenated fats. Many fat-containing processed foods in the UK still only list the main types of fat, i.e. total saturated and unsaturated fat, without specifying the individual types which may have a high linoleate content. Some of the more socially responsible food companies are now marketing fat containing products labelled as containing no partially hydrogenated vegetable oil, i.e. containing no ITFs.

Hydrogenated fats can play a significant role in the development of obesity. When a meal containing high levels of glucose is eaten, insulin is released into the blood stream from the pancreas. Insulin induces an increase in cell surface receptors which bind to glucose and transport it into cells for storage and this is a completely normal process. Many of the molecules involved in these glucose and insulin mediated pathways are fatty acids. An increased level of dietary ITF can make the cellular membrane stiffer and stickier, which inhibits the glucose transport mechanism. As a result, more glucose remains in the blood stream. This results in increased insulin production by the pancreas in an attempt to lower the blood glucose level. The excess insulin causes an increase in lipogenesis, the insulin mediated conversion of glucose into TGs. This elevated serum TG is deposited in adipose cells throughout the body, particularly as abdominal fat.

Partially hydrogenated fats (ITF-containing) are deposited in body fat and can increase the risk of breast cancer development in women [101, 106]. Partially hydrogenated fats can increase the risk for heart attack by raising blood levels of lipoprotein (a) (Lpa) to cause artery blocking [107, 108] and also by lowering blood omega-3 fat activity [109]. Babies and infants do not escape the effects of ITFs. Studies show that partially hydrogenated fats may slow growth and development in infants [110]. ITFs have also been shown to stimulate several other processes associated with increased risk of CHD. Interestingly, the omega-3 fats can reverse most of the damaging effects of ITFs (see Table 5). These data indicate just how crucial omega-3 fats are in healthy diets. No single pharmaceutical product (e.g. statins) could ever replace omega-3 fats for optimum protection against heart disease and perhaps even some cancers.

Finally, to avoid any future confusion the trans fat problem needs to be clarified. Legislation now decrees that the ITF content of foods should be clearly labelled. This means that dairy products will now have their trans fat content listed. However, the natural trans fats derived from cow's milk are readily metabolised, unlike the toxic vegetable oil-derived ITFs.

More enlightened sections of the oils and fats industry are moving away from the old trans fat yielding processes. The problem of solidifying oils is being addressed by using a process called interesterification, which uses enzymes to exchange fatty acids between different oils and solid fats, resulting in hybrid fats with appropriate melting points. The process of interesterification

Table 5 **Health effects of omega-3 fats and industrial trans fats**

Long chain omega-3 fats	Industrial trans fats
Lower LDL cholesterol	Raise LDL cholesterol
Raise HDL cholesterol	Lower HDL cholesterol
Lower blood fat in post-prandial lipaemia (in high doses)	Raise blood fat and cause obesity
Anti-inflammatory activity	Stimulate inflammatory activity by activating the TNF system [a]
Inhibit platelet aggregation and cell adhesion involved in plaque formation	
Improve endothelial cell function to lower blood pressure	Impair endothelial cell function to cause reduction in brachial artery vasodilation which increases blood pressure
Reduce plaque formation	Increase plaque formation by raising plasma Lpa levels to form 'sticky' LDL
Reduce insulin insensitivity to improve glucose response in Syndrome X and diabetic patients	Modify cell membrane receptor responses to increase insulin insensitivity, impairing the glucose reponse in these patients
In 31 randomised controlled trials dietary omega-3 fats lowered CVD mortality by an average of 32%	7 large epidemiological studies have shown that a 2% increase in dietary energy intake as ITFs was associated with a 29% increase in the incidence of CVD
Reduce arterial calcification	

[a] TNF (tumour necrosis factor) is a crucial component of the body's defence against cancer. However, if it is stimulated inappropriately it can give rise to a damaging inflammatory response.

does not, however, address the problems of rancidity which will probably require the addition of natural antioxidants, or the problems of excessive linoleate (omega-6) in the new hybrid fats. Very recent research indicates that interesterified fats may not be the best replacement for hydrogenated fats as they appear to have similar effects as the ITFs on insulin and cholesterol levels.

It is now possible to seek out food products that are labelled as containing no hydrogenated fat. Recent US legislation limits ITF content in food to a maximum of 500mg per portion, resulting in some companies reducing the portion size to just under 500mg, and the ITF content does not need to be specified.

In response to adverse opinion about industrial trans fats and health, Monsanto, Du Pont and others have increased massively the production of low-linolenic soybeans in the US from 600,000 to 1.8 million acres, but this does not address the issue of excessive amounts of linoleate in popular cooking oils.

The US and UK support for freedom of choice relies on public awareness of nutrition problems and the commitment to scrutinising food labels. It is probably unrealistic to expect the general public to spend a lot of time interpreting complicated food labels (often on the back of the packaging in extremely small print). The Danish government has decided, on the basis of recent research, to limit the ITF content of fats to less than 2%. Hopefully the health benefits of this legislation will be seen during the next decade.

The low fat diet myth

It is a common belief that saturated fat in particular and too much fat in general is bad for health. As a result, many people have tried to reduce the amount of fat they consume. This has led to in a rise in the consumption of refined carbohydrate and can be correlated with a rise in the incidence of certain chronic diseases and obesity. We respond by modifying our diet to eat the amount of calories that make us feel satisfied and will support our daily energy requirements. As the low fat diet myth has been gradually propagated throughout society, we have all gradually increased our consumption of carbohydrates to replace the energy lost from consuming less fat.

Recent research has indicated that low fat diets result in the oxidation and depletion of the essential omega-3 fats. These cardio-protective fats are already at a sub optimal concentration in such diets. Data relating to the initial incidence of heart disease is extremely difficult to find, the accent being on palliative treatment, which shows sustained improvement. However, primary diagnosis in the UK shows a continued increase despite the stabilisation of fat consumption.

Fat provides more calories per g [48] than sugar or protein [59]. Low fat cookies, yoghurts or ready prepared slimmer's meals are invariably high in carbohydrates. So if carbohydrate is substituted for fat weight for weight in the diet, fewer calories are consumed. Contrary to the wisdom of some diet schemes, this has no real benefit for people wishing to slim or maintain a healthy diet. Hunger, and therefore the amount of food consumed, is triggered by low blood sugar and the emptiness of the stomach. Food rich in fat tends to remain in the stomach longer than carbohydrates. Understanding how to combat hunger is far more beneficial to slimming and a healthy diet than calorie counting. Hunger is effectively reduced by modifying the diet to increase the digestion time. This is because the human digestive system has evolved to release rapidly every available calorie from nutrient-poor diets. The feeling of hunger following a high protein/fat meal returns much more slowly because fat and protein are digested more slowly and remain in the stomach longer. A high fat/protein meal induces only a minimal rise in blood sugar and insulin release from the pancreas, thus avoiding the food cravings associated with the insulin release cycle. In addition, fibre rich fruit, vegetables and salads add bulk to the diet and extend digestion time, resulting in a controlled release of nutrients into the digestive system.

Meals high in fat and protein also promote the release of glucagon, rather than insulin, from the pancreas [111]. Glucagon maintains the blood glucose concentration by stimulating the liver to release glucose from the glycogen stores. It also promotes the breaking down of body fat for several hours after the meal is eaten and inhibits the synthesis of fatty acids in fat stores. This benefits those wishing to slim.

Dietary change and the obesity epidemic

Obesity in America, which remained constant through the 1960s and early 1970s, has surged from 13% of the population in the early 1970s to over 35% today (see Figure 5). During this same period, there has been a change in the consumption of fats, and a 6% reduction in the proportion of calories they provide in our diets. Whilst the *percentage* of fat in the diet has decreased, the *actual amount* of fat consumed remained fairly constant (Figure 7). This may sound contradictory, but means that people are consuming more carbohydrate without reducing fat intake. This suggests that the obesity epidemic is a consequence of people obtaining more of their calories from refined carbohydrates, particularly sugar. The increased consumption of partially hydrogenated vegetable oils is also of crucial importance, because these products contain high levels of trans fats and linoleate which are known to stimulate fat accumulation [112].

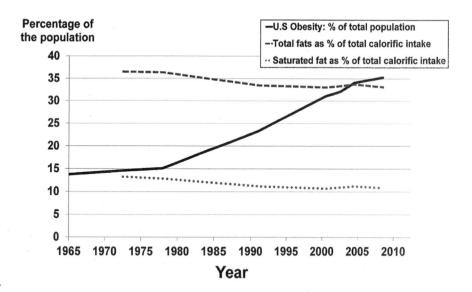

Figure 5 Trends in fat consumption and obesity in the U.S.A.

Figure 5 shows a sharp inflection at or around 1980 in the incidence of obesity. This coincides with a massive increase in the production and consumption of fast foods containing the dangerous combination of salt, refined carbohydrate, omega-6 fat and ITFs, due to deregulation in the food industry with replacement of animal fats by vegetable oils, and replacement of sucrose with high fructose syrup in fizzy drinks. Moreover, at around the same time, the sweetener aspartame was cleared for use as a drinks additive. In addition to its several toxic effects, aspartame has been shown to increase cravings for sweet foods and is largely useless as a slimming aid.

Simply controlling calorific intake may not be the healthy answer to weight loss. The type of food consumed appears to be more important. It is simpler to maintain a healthy body weight by modifying the type of food eaten rather than periodic bouts of calorie counting. Many calorie controlled diets have poor long-term outcomes because when the calorie counting stops, the weight is usually regained.

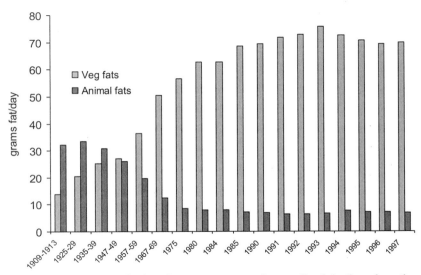

***Figure 6* Trends in the consumption of added animal and vegetable fats in the U.S.A.**

The actual changes in fat consumption from 1909 to 1997 are shown in Figure 6. Note the massive proportional increase in vegetable fat intake (ITF-rich) from 1957 to 1979. This precedes the inflection in the adult obesity curve seen in 1980 (Figure 5). This sudden inflection may be due to the young adults, raised on a high vegetable fat diet for 20 years, being subjected to high carbohydrate/fat diets from the late 1970s onwards. In 1950 fat consumption was about 50g/day, with equal proportions of vegetable and animal fat. By 1980, fat consumption had risen by some 35% with animal fat taking up less than 10% of the total (Figure 6).

The increase in total fat consumption in the first half of the 20th century arose from increases in the consumption of margarines, vegetable oils and shortening, which replaced animal fats, butter and lard. This resulted in an increased proportion of ITFs and linoleate in the diet, further exacerbated by increased

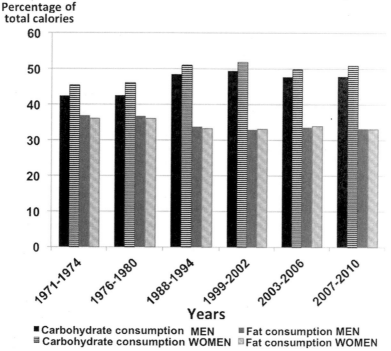

Percentage of total calories

■ Carbohydrate consumption MEN   ■ Fat consumption MEN
▤ Carbohydrate consumption WOMEN   ▨ Fat consumption WOMEN

Figure 7 **Trends in fat and carbohydrate consumption in the U.S.A.**

95

consumption of processed foods in the 1980s. We propose that this led to the profoundly unhealthy dietary combination of highly refined carbohydrates (Figure 4), and omega-6 fats and ITFs (Figure 6), which may account for the startling increase in obesity (see Figure 5), and its associated diseases.

The effect of these dietary changes in the late 1970s may have been compounded by the development of computer games, watching TV and other sedentary activity. Very recently a UK study has linked childhood obesity with lack of sleep causing stress which leads to overeating.

Effect of high fat diets on health

Many human populations can consume large amounts of fat and remain perfectly healthy. The Masai have existed for the past 10,000 years as cattle-herding nomads in East Africa. Their diet was mainly derived from large amounts of high fat milk and meat. Masai males used to eat up to 300g of mainly saturated fat per day. The indigenous Masai have been recorded as having one of the lowest average cholesterol levels ever measured. Autopsies on Masai males showed an almost complete absence of the atherosclerotic lesions implicated in coronary heart disease. Their extremely active lifestyle also made a crucial contribution to their health, spectacular physiques and lack of obesity.

Another East African tribe, the Samburus, had an even higher fat intake than the Masai. The Samburu males consumed up to 400g of animal fat daily. The Samburus displayed both low total serum cholesterol levels and an absence of heart disease [113]. Numerous other examples conflict with the idea that fat consumption causes heart disease. Interestingly, it has been observed that when populations such as the Masai migrate to other areas where refined sugary foods are consumed, together with a less active lifestyle, their LDL cholesterol levels rise.

Studies have shown that the French have the lowest incidence of heart disease in the Western world, whilst consuming the highest level of saturated fat. Specifically, the French have a 10% higher blood cholesterol than Americans, but a 25% lower incidence of heart disease. This is commonly referred to as the French paradox [114]. More surprising is the Spanish paradox. Studies in 1995 and 2003 showed that heart disease fell by 25% in men and 34% in women following a 50% drop in carbohydrate consumption and the adoption of a high animal fat/protein diet. These data suggest that neither high nor low blood cholesterol levels are predictive of heart disease. The traditional Inuit diet also demonstrates the value of a fat-rich diet. Their diet rich in polyunsaturated fat protected them against heart disease and cancer. Once they moved on to hamburgers, cola, ice cream and doughnuts, these benefits were lost.

Dietary fat and heart disease: is there really a link?

The notion that dietary fat makes you fat and fat causes heart disease is the common belief of the majority of the general public and many medical practitioners. As a result, the rush to reduce total fat intake in our diets has encouraged a shift to highly refined carbohydrate diets, which actually increase our risk of developing heart disease, diabetes, obesity and many cancers.

The common sense notion that fatty deposits in the heart must be a consequence of eating too much fat is highly questionable when we look at the available scientific evidence. It appears that the human body can manage the metabolism of fat very effectively.

The first piece of evidence in support of the theory that consumption of fat causes heart disease was presented by Russian researchers in the first part of the 20th century. The researchers caused fatty deposits to build up in rabbit arteries by feeding them large amounts of animal fats, and cholesterol was blamed for these deposits [115]. However, these experiments were only successful in herbivorous animals, animals whose digestive system is not designed to digest meat, animal fat or cholesterol. Similar experiments with carnivorous animals failed to induce fatty deposit build-up in the arteries of the animals [116]. As we are omnivorous and capable of eating meat, these experiments have little relevance to our health concerns.

A common argument used in support of a link between fat consumption and heart disease is that countries with high dietary levels of saturated animal fat have high levels of heart disease. This is undoubtedly true, but individuals in these countries also have the highest consumption of sugar, refined carbohydrates, polyunsaturated vegetable oils, hydrogenated vegetable oils and the lowest levels of physical activity. All of these factors have been implicated in the development of heart disease. For a convincing argument in favour of the idea that fat consumption leads to the development of heart disease, we need more than the currently available circumstantial and anecdotal evidence.

In 1988 the US Surgeon General's Office initiated an investigative report on the dangers of dietary fat. After 11 years and an expenditure of 17 million dollars, the project was abandoned in June 1999. This report was initiated with the preconceived idea that it would find that dietary fat played a significant role in the elevation of blood cholesterol and the development of heart disease. The project was unable to find conclusive proof. It turns out that the relationship between dietary fat and disease is not nearly as simple as it once appeared.

Role of blood lipids in heart disease

Normally a fasting blood sample will be requested to obtain baseline values for blood lipids and proteins, unaffected by recent meals, upon which a diagnosis will be made. However, with respect to blood lipids, recent research has demonstrated that the patients' response to dietary lipids and their clearance from the plasma is a far more important predictor of heart disease risk than fasting plasma lipid levels. The impaired clearance of lipids from the blood following a fatty meal is referred to as post-prandial lipaemia (PPL), and is now thought to be a major risk factor in the initiation and progression of atherosclerosis.

Next time you visit your GP to have a cholesterol measurement taken in an attempt to assess your general health and the risk of developing coronary heart disease, make sure that you have the results for both HDL and LDL cholesterol, and that you also ask for a lipoprotein (a) measurement to be taken. In addition one could include homocysteine and C-reactive protein tests, which are potent indicators of heart disease risk. If you have an apparently slim build, and a family history of heart disease, it would be wise to request a blood leptin test as well, to reveal whether or not you have 'hidden' abdominal fat which is closely linked with heart disease. Finally a blood lipid clearance test following a fatty meal can reveal PPL and the need for remedial fish oil consumption.

99

Post-prandial lipaemia in long-term cardiovascular health and diabetes

The healthy response to the digestion of a fatty meal is for the blood lipid levels to rise and then fall quite sharply when the chylomicrons are rapidly depleted of TGs, which are transferred to HDL and LDL particles. The cholesterol-rich remnant chylomicron particles are then taken up by liver receptors and further metabolised.

In PPL patients, the depletion of TGs from the chylomicrons is sluggish and the TG-rich remnant particles are only weakly bound by the liver receptors. These particles persist in the blood where they release TGs for uptake by HDL and LDL. The TAG-rich HDL and LDL are then degraded by a hepatic lipase to yield small, dense HDL and LDL. The small dense HDL are rapidly degraded, leading to a drop in the plasma HDL concentration. However, the small dense LDL are not degraded and may become oxidised and taken up by macrophages to form foam cells which drive the process of atherogenesis (see Appendix).

The condition of PPL appears to have a genetic basis where it is referred to as the Atherogenic Lipoprotein Phenotype, and there is a strong association between this condition and Metabolic Syndrome. Some of the characteristics of PPL are shown in Table 6.

Several recent studies have shown that men with high plasma TGs and low HDL concentrations have a twofold to threefold risk of developing ischaemic heart disease. In addition, the extent of atherosclerosis is increased by continued exposure to TG-rich remnant particles. The inherited condition of impaired

TG tolerance in PPL is now recognised as a major predisposing factor in arterial disease.

Dietary fish oils can lower TAG blood levels resulting from PPL

The typical elevation of plasma TG in PPL is most commonly seen in diets which are rich in saturated, monounsaturated and omega-6 PUFAs. By contrast, meals containing adequate amounts of omega-3 fish oils have the effect of reducing PPL. Long-term diets containing around 2g/day of long chain omega-3 fats from fish oils have resulted in the reduction of PPL by 30% [117]. Although this is encouraging news for susceptible patients, it will require a tenfold increase in the consumption of fish oil when the average UK consumption is around 0.2g per day.

Dietary fat, obesity and cancer

Cancer is more common in obese individuals. Many groups have used this fact to suggest falsely that as dietary fat makes us fat, then dietary fat must cause cancer. This is incorrect, and as always the devil is in the detail. Consumption of fat alone does not make us fat; what makes us fat is the consumption of excess

Table 6 **Exaggerated post-prandial lipaemia**

Raised fasting TAGs (≥1.5mM)

Presence of small dense LDL

Reduced fasting HDL cholesterol (≤1mM)

Reduced proportion of large HDL

Increased presence of cholesterol ester-rich chylomicron remnant particles

Insulin resistance

---

calories. In modern Western diets, carbohydrates are the biggest contributors to excess calorie consumption, and therefore obesity, and the associated increased risk of cancer.

Cancer is more prevalent in the obese

A 16 year study in the US involving 900,000 people suggested that death rates from all cancers combined in clinically obese individuals was 52% higher for men and 62% higher for women than the rates in men and women of normal weight. In both men and women, obesity was significantly associated with higher rates of death due to cancer of the oesophagus, colon, rectum, liver, gallbladder, pancreas and kidney. Significant trends of increasing risk with increasing obesity were observed for death from cancers of the stomach and prostate in men and for death from cancers of the breast, uterus, cervix and ovary in women. On the basis of these results, the authors suggested that 14% of all deaths from cancer in men and 20% of all deaths from cancer in women in the US were attributed to being overweight and obesity [118]. Given the evidence that supports the role of sugar, ITFs and overconsumption of linoleate in the incidence of obesity, this places a huge burden of responsibility on food corporations.

Dietary advice

Storage of omega-3 rich oils

Foods containing these essential polyunsaturated fats must be consumed fresh and not stored at room temperature, as these fats rapidly oxidise in air and become rancid, forming potentially toxic peroxides. These oils are typically cold pressed under inert gas and best refrigerated in an airtight container away from light. The alternative is to obtain fresh seeds and nuts and consume them as soon as possible. Fish oils (e.g. cod liver oil) should also be deep frozen and used quickly, unless they are bought as gelatine capsules, which have a shelf life of several weeks.

Vegetable oils that can be healthily consumed, stored at room temperature and used for cooking are rapeseed, palm and coconut oils. Olive oil, particularly extra virgin oil, is best used as a salad dressing and not in cooking, as it has a low smoking temperature and can become oxidised. If you are not a vegetarian, lard, butter and ghee are healthy alternatives, particularly for frying. When frying a good tip is to emulate the Chinese and add a small amount of water to the wok or frying pan. This lowers the frying temperature to 100°C, lowers the amount of fat required, and reduces the amount of oxidative damage which normally occurs in high temperature fat frying.

Recent developments in the vegetable oil industry

Monsanto, Du Pont and some other companies are developing new strains of soybean enriched with stearidonic acid which is converted to EPA more efficiently in the body, requiring only a fourfold excess. This is an extremely important development as increasing demand for omega-3 fish oils will put more pressure on supplies of oily fish.

A diet containing polyunsaturated fats must contain adequate antioxidant vitamins and minerals to protect these oxygen-sensitive fat compounds.

Toxicity of ITFs and rancid oils/oils used for cooking

One should avoid hydrogenated oils found in processed foods and margarines, as well as the partially hydrogenated supermarket polyunsaturated vegetable oils, such as sunflower oil, because they are contaminated with ITFs, as are most commercial salad dressings (see Chapter 7). These oils are often advertised as being rich in polyunsaturates, but they are in the wrong ratios because they have been chemically treated to prevent rancidity. In the process of hydrogenation, the essential omega-3 fats are reduced to omega-6 fats, high levels of which have unhealthy side effects.

Some of the most dangerous products which should be avoided are vegetarian suet, which contains as much as 25% trans fat, and the hard margarines (15–20% ITFs). Many chefs will tell you that these products are perfect for pastry baking, but are unaware of their unhealthy properties.

Pure polyunsaturated fats, those obtained from fresh whole foods like nuts and fresh fish, however, are good for our health. Certain nuts and seeds and oily fish contain beneficial levels of these polyunsaturated fats. It is important to realise that polyunsaturated fats go rancid quickly, when they have been processed into oils, so foods rich in polyunsaturated fats should be used quickly and fresh supplies bought regularly. If possible these foods and oils should be refrigerated and the oils should not be used for cooking because the high temperatures greatly accelerate the speed at which these healthy oils become peroxidised and very toxic. Once polyunsaturated fats have peroxidised, they lose their health giving qualities and actually become toxic. It is worth knowing that when polyunsaturated fats have peroxidised, they taste bitter. This is particularly noticeable in the case of walnuts, walnut oil and cod liver oil, which become bitter tasting and toxic if kept too long.

Healthy alternatives

We should not strive to replace saturated fats completely in our diet with polyunsaturated fats. Indeed, the supposedly healthy option of polyunsaturated fats must certainly be used with caution, particularly with respect to partially hydrogenated vegetable oils which contain ITFs. Monounsaturated fats like olive oil and canola (rapeseed) oil, and saturated fats such as coconut oil and palm oil are good alternatives to the polyunsaturated oils and are more stable in cooking. Butter is a stable fat, comprised largely of short and medium chain fatty acids, which are easily broken down and used by the body. Butter, ghee (clarified butter) olive oil, palm oil and coconut oil can be heated when cooking, but only gently and not to excess.

Finally we should stress moderation in diet as in all things. Just because fresh PUFAs are essential for health does not mean that they should be consumed to excess. Overconsumption of PUFAs can lead to an increase in oxidative stress in the body, a condition caused by the depletion of vitamin E used up to scavenge free radicals formed from the excessive levels of oxygen-sensitive PUFAs. This condition has been implicated in the causes of heart disease and cancer. Leading edge research now indicates that ITFs and omega-6 PUFAs are the predominant risk factors rather than animal fats. A recent dietary study in the US with 50,000 patients has shown that animal fat is not a risk factor. If one wanted to supplement one's diet with PUFAs, then this would be best done in conjunction with a good source of natural vitamin E, the best choice being wheat germ oil.

The omega-3, omega-6 fat controversy

There is now overwhelming evidence that supports the need for adequate levels of long chain omega-3 fats, EPA and DHA, in the diet. They are obtained mainly from fish oils and have been shown to play a vital role in the maintenance of a healthy heart and circulation, infant brain development, visual acuity and cognitive function in the elderly.

Currently, there is an important debate taking place between the European Food Standards Authority (EFSA), the food industry and concerned lipid scientists, which mirrors the problems revealed in the WHO sugar debate (see Chapter 3). It concerns serious flaws in the ESFA-recommended omega-3 dietary reference values (DRVs), now legitimised in EEU guidelines for food labelling. Rather than the inclusion of preformed long chain omega-3 fats, EPA and DHA, from fish oils, the use of the much cheaper short chain, plant-based omega-3 fats is to be sanctioned. It appears that the EFSA have based their dietary proposals on advice from the food industry. Basic research has clearly shown that dietary EPA and DHA confer substantial health benefits and are best obtained from a diet rich in oily fish. Vegetarians obtain their EPA and DHA from dietary α-linolenate but the conversion rate is very poor. However, they tend not to consume excessive amounts of processed foods that are rich in omega-6. Synthesis of 1g of the long chain omega-3 acid mixture would require the consumption of some 14g of α-linolenate, even under optimum dietary conditions.

With the omega-6:omega-3 ratios reaching 10:1 in the UK and nearer to 20:1 in the US, the inclusion of plant-based, short chain omega-3 fats in food products would appear to have insignificant health benefits, due to the diluting-out effects of the high concentrations of dietary omega-6 fats from processed foods and vegetable oils. Furthermore, the EFSA has specified a much lower daily recommended intake level of 250mg/day of EPA + DHA. An expert panel of 22 scientists together with government research laboratories and several international research groups propose a daily intake of at least 500mg/day. In dietary terms, this could comprise the following options:

- Two portions of oily fish per week

- 2×1g fish oil capsules per day containing 500–600mg of EPA + DHA

- 7g of α-linolenate/day from flax oil or other plant sources (2 tsps) algal sources of EPA + DHA to yield 500mg/day.

An equivalent intake of the omega-6 fatty acid linoleate, would give an optimum 1:1 ratio seen in the traditional Inuit diets. This would require an extremely large reduction in the consumption of linoleate-rich vegetable fats. The consumption of these fats has risen by a staggering 1,000-fold since 1945 [119]. This is due to the massive expansion of the oil seed industry which produces the omega-6 (linoleate) rich oils such as corn, soybean and sunflower oils that have largely replaced dietary animal fats (Table 7, Figure 7).

Our grandparents' generation consumed a saturated fat-rich diet (40% of total calories) supplemented with milligram quantities of omega-6 and omega-3 fats, mainly from meat and fish. We are now consuming gram quantities of linoleate from these vegetable oils, but our consumption of omega-3 oil at 0.2g/day is less than half the recommended amount.

The combined effects of trans fat intake and linoleate overconsumption must surely be a crucial factor in the development of inflammatory diseases since the Second World War. Recent studies on US mortality figures indicate that low dietary omega-3 fat coupled with excessive omega-6 intake may be responsible for at least 100,000 deaths per annum.

Table 7 **Percentage fatty acid content of edible oils and fats**

Dietary fat	Saturated	Omega-6	Omega-3	Mono-unsaturated
Safflower	10	76	1	14
Sunflower	12	71	1	16
Corn	13	67	1	29
Soybean	15	54	8	23
Cottonseed	27	54	1	19
Peanut	19	33	0.5	48
Canola (rape)	7	21	11	61
Flaxseed	9	16	57	18
Palm	51	10	1	39
Olive	15	9	1	75
Beef tallow	48	2	1	49
Lard	43	9	1	47
Butterfat	68	3	1	28
Coconut	91	2	0	7

This problem should be addressed by a large reduction in the intake of fats rich in linoleate fats, with a more modest twofold increase in omega-3 intake. For example, omitting the first six oils in Table 7 from the diet will achieve a substantial reduction in linoleate uptake. Processed foods containing vegetable oils should be avoided, and oily fish should be eaten at least twice a week. Cod liver oil is a good source of EPA and DHA and also contains vitamin D which is crucial for bone development and maintenance.

The term omega-3 fatty acid on food packaging is too unspecific and misleading. The most important thing is to look for the abbreviations EPA and DHA, which stand for the essential long chain omega-3 fatty acids derived from fish oil or algae. Plant derived, short chain omega-3 fatty acids like α-linolenic acid when added to foods and dietary supplements will not confer appropriate health benefits unless consumed in larger quantities.

Many health food shops and supermarkets are now selling foods supplemented with plant based omega-3, omega-6 and omega-9 fatty acids. Omega-9 is non essential in our diet, omega-6 is already in excess in the diet and plant omega-3 is very poorly converted into the health-promoting EPA and DHA.

Conclusions: healthy and unhealthy fats

Data presented in this chapter has been sourced from some of the best laboratories and research groups from the past 50 years, and has received general acceptance from the scientific community. After prolonged publicity, the food companies have recently accepted that ITFs are a dietary health risk and are searching for safe alternatives. However, there is still confusion over the health risks of excessive consumption of linoleate-rich vegetable oils, the deficiency of omega-3 fat in the diet, and the value of interesterification as a replacement for the hydrogenation process.

Many in the medical profession are comfortable with the current high levels of linoleate in the diet because of its purported health benefits in lowering LDL cholesterol. This notion will be further challenged in the next chapter.

Publicity in the popular press and advisory medical bulletins to reduce saturated fat consumption is too simplistic. Rather, one should eat a calorie-controlled diet in which saturated or monounsaturated fat is the major lipid energy source. The intake of omega-6 or linoleate containing fats should be greatly reduced by restricting the consumption of vegetable oils and processed foods which have a high omega-6 content. The daily requirement for omega-3 fat requires a modest increase in the consumption of oily fish (two times a week) or fish oil capsules (once a day). Vegetarians can obtain adequate omega-3 fat from about two teaspoons of flax oil per day. Finally, sufficient dietary fat is required to allow the uptake of essential oil-soluble vitamins and pigments.

6   Cholesterol, essential for health

In the US, hundreds of millions of dollars have been
spent on studies to try to identify a connection
between cholesterol and heart disease, and these have
all failed. It is a fact that half of the people with heart
disease have normal cholesterol levels. The only
concrete connection between cholesterol and heart
disease risk is among people with hypercholesterolaemia, a genetic disease characterised by pathol-
ogically high blood cholesterol. Some processed food
industries are responding to public and media
pressure by reducing the amount of ITFs in their
products. The food oil producers are moving swiftly to
engineer new strains with oil composition that does
not require hydrogenation, but a reduction in the
omega-6 linoleate content appears not to be a priority.
High sugar intake is linked to high LDL cholesterol,
serum TGs and increased risk of CVD.

Introduction

Cholesterol is found in animal meat and fish, milk, eggs and dairy
products and belongs to a class of natural compounds called
sterols, found only in animal tissues. Cholesterol plays a vital role
in cell membrane structure, and is also a precursor for bile acids,
sex hormones and other natural steroid hormones. In the absence
of dietary cholesterol it can be synthesised in the liver from
carbohydrate or fat. Cholesterol and its esters attached to long
chain fatty acids are extremely insoluble in water and have to be
transported in the blood inside lipoprotein vesicles or particles.

Lipoprotein transport and metabolism

Large lipoprotein particles called chylomicrons appear in the blood only after a fatty meal. They are formed in the intestinal cells and contain cholesterol, its esters and a large excess of triacylglycerol (TG). They transport TGs to all the tissues of the body, in the process becoming cholesterol-rich, TG-depleted remnant chylomicrons. These remnant particles then enter the liver and release their cholesterol, which is incorporated into very low density lipoproteins (VLDLs). In the absence of dietary cholesterol and TG, the liver synthesises these lipids and incorporates them into the VLDLs. The VLDLs then enter the blood and deliver TGs to the tissues to become remnants which become intermediate density lipoproteins (IDLs). The IDLs can then either re-enter the liver or pick up cholesterol from high density lipoproteins (HDLs) to form low density lipoproteins (LDLs). LDLs are the major source of cholesterol for the non-hepatic tissues. HDLs are first formed as protein-rich particles in the liver. They enter the blood and scavenge cholesterol from the tissues, chylomicrons and VLDL remnants, convert it to its esters and then transport cholesterol and its esters back to the liver.

Historical perspectives

In 1900 a research team in Germany identified a 'sticky' form of LDL cholesterol in human atherosclerotic plaques, areas of artery wall containing fatty deposits that can be responsible for heart attacks. The stickiness was caused by lipoprotein (a) in the LDL particles [120]. The significance of this substance was largely discounted until recently, when a re-evaluation of the 50 year Framingham Heart Study indicated that lipoprotein (a) is a better indicator in predicting heart disease than the normally used LDL/HDL ratio or total cholesterol level.

Many in the scientific community and general public still believe that cholesterol is the major risk factor in CVD. This arises, in part, from research carried out more than half a century ago. Rabbits were fed a high cholesterol diet and developed atherosclerotic plaques in their arteries. Clearly, cholesterol is not a component in natural rabbit food and when the same experiments were carried out using carnivorous animals, the results were negative. No increase in plaque formation was seen. The negative experiments were not widely reported. More recently, experiments by the Nobel Prize winners Brown and Goldstein revealed a link between cholesterol and heart disease, but only in patients with the genetic disease known as familial hypercholesterolaemia which is characterised by excessively high blood cholesterol levels.

Nobody was really worried about the health aspects of cholesterol until about 25 years ago. The outcome of a study concerning the relationship between heart disease, cholesterol and dietary fats led to guidelines in the US for reducing consumption of eggs, butter and most other animal fats that may play a role in altering cholesterol levels. The study's recommendation was based on the hypothesis that cholesterol causes heart disease because a large proportion of individuals with heart complaints had high cholesterol.

The functions of LDL and HDL have been outlined because knowledge of what these terms mean is extremely useful when trying to understand the role of cholesterol in health. The situation is now becoming further complicated as VLDL and chylomicron remnants are also being proposed as agents in arterial dysfunction. LDL is often referred to as 'bad cholesterol' due to its high concentrations of cholesterol esters and TGs and an association with increased risk of heart disease. HDL is often

113

referred to as 'good cholesterol' and has been associated with a reduced risk of heart disease. The terms 'good' and 'bad' should be used with caution because LDL particles play a vital role in delivering cholesterol to growing cells, where it is incorporated as an essential membrane component and to the organs and tissues where steroid hormones are synthesised. LDLs only become a risk factor when they are produced in excess of the body's requirements, and become oxidised during vascular inflammation. LDLs per se are not harmful. In fact, a high blood LDL concentration is crucial in infant development for delivering adequate cholesterol and TGs to growing tissues.

Excessively high LDL levels in adults present a risk because of the increased amount of cholesterol available for oxidation to 7-oxocholesterol by free radicals generated by oxidative stress, which in turn is stimulated by mental and physical stress, inflammation, lack of exercise and an antioxidant deficient diet. This process occurs not in the blood but between the vessel lining or endothelium and the smooth muscle wall, in the intima. LDLs migrate from the blood into the intima. Under oxidative stress, they become damaged by free radicals known as reactive oxygen species (ROS). A complex series of events then occurs which can lead to narrowing of the arteries and eventually blockage (see Appendix for further details).

The level of each type of cholesterol is a more accurate indicator of heart disease risk than measuring total blood cholesterol. The current method of assessing risk of developing heart disease is to estimate the amount of LDL and HDL in the blood. A high level of LDL and low level of HDL would indicate a higher risk of developing heart disease, whilst high HDL and low LDL levels lessen the risk of developing heart disease.

Dietary fat, cholesterol and heart disease

It is an oversimplification to blame dietary saturated fat for causing coronary heart disease. The results of studies concerning saturated fat and heart disease are often contradictory, inconclusive and ambiguous [121]. The widespread notion that saturated fat raises LDL cholesterol and is a major risk factor in CHD arises from several flawed studies, where fat intake was not corrected for the presence of industrial trans fats (ITFs) and the pro-inflammatory omega-6 fatty acid linoleate. Earlier studies on the naturally high animal fat diets of the Masai and Inuit showed a negligible incidence of CHD, but of course their diets did not contain any ITFs. A recent review of 12 randomised controlled trials has demonstrated that dietary ITFs raise LDL cholesterol, lower HDL cholesterol and increase the ratio of total cholesterol to HDL cholesterol.

Effects of saturated fatty acids on the total cholesterol concentration, LDL/HDL ratio and postprandial lipaemia

Several hours after a meal containing fat, the plasma TG level rises. This is a normal response and is referred to as postprandial lipaemia. However, if the plasma TG level rises too high, it is associated with an increased risk of heart disease. One of the mechanisms involved is the activation of factor VIII which is involved in blood clotting. Different saturated fatty acids have different effects on postprandial lipaemia. It is raised by palmitic acid and lowered by stearic acid which also lowers the activation of factor VIII. These effects appear to be related to the melting points of the fatty acids. Increasing carbon chain length raises the melting point of the fat. For example, taking palmitic acid, with 16 carbon atoms, and stearic acid, with 18 carbon atoms, fat rich

115

in stearic acid will have a higher melting point than fat rich in palmitic acid, with the more solid fat being protective [121].

Recent investigations have used the total cholesterol/HDL cholesterol ratio to examine the role of dietary fatty acids in modifying both LDL and HDL levels. An analysis of 60 controlled studies has shown that stearic acid lowers LDL cholesterol levels, and HDL cholesterol levels either remain steady or are raised [123]. Recent research has suggested that stearic acid is the healthiest replacement for ITFs in products where a solid fat is required. Beef fat contains a mixture of 50% stearic and oleic acids, and is a much healthier alternative to the high-linoleate vegetable oils.

Studies in the 1990s have indicated that a reduction in consumption of fat and particularly saturated fat led to a decrease in the proportion of HDL in the blood, thus potentially increasing the risk of heart disease [124, 125]. Contrary to popular belief, evidence is mounting that refutes the link between the consumption of saturated fat and heart disease.

What can be done to raise the level of HDL cholesterol? Strangely enough, only two things; exercise and eating fat [126]. Actually, all fats will raise HDL levels, but some saturated fats will raise HDL more than others [127, 128]. Most saturated fats, with minor exceptions, do not raise total blood cholesterol levels [129, 130]. In conclusion it appears that consuming saturated fats is not a problem for healthy, active individuals.

If we reduce our intake of saturated fat in an attempt to reduce our cholesterol levels, where will we get the calories that were provided by fat? The calories derived from fat will be replaced, if not from protein, by calories derived from carbohydrates and sugar. This is a far more dangerous situation in terms of heart disease. Carbohydrates and sugar raise insulin which stimulates serum LDL cholesterol and TG synthesis, and together with lower HDL generally increase inflammation, heart disease risk, cancer and increased mortality [131–134].

In 2000, a study was performed to determine the effects of variations in dietary fat and carbohydrate consumption upon levels of TGs in the blood (a high level of TGs being a risk factor for heart disease) in eight healthy, non-diabetic volunteers. The results suggested that carbohydrates led to an increase in TG levels; hence the wisdom of the recommendation that we should replace dietary saturated fat with carbohydrates is questionable [135]. The few studies that indicate a correlation between saturated fat and cholesterol reduction and a lower risk of CHD also clearly document an increase in deaths from cancer, suicide, violence and brain haemorrhage [136].

Replacement of ITFs in processed foods

Now that the toxic effects of ITFs have been clearly demonstrated, their total replacement in processed foods is an urgent priority. The food oil companies are striving to modify the oil seed plants in order to lower their polyunsaturated fatty acid (PUFA) content and eliminate the need for hydrogenation. Considerable success has been achieved with the production of low-PUFA soybean and sunflower strains. However, some of the strains are the product of genetic manipulation rather than traditional cross-breeding, and may meet market resistance, particularly in Europe. The original solution to the problem was simply to replace ITFs with saturated fatty acids with the appropriate physical properties such as a higher melting point for margarine production. The reality is more complex.

Other CVD risk factors

Other factors have a major influence upon the potential of developing heart disease. Certain lifestyle habits such as smoking, lack of exercise and the excessive consumption of refined carbohydrate foods have all been associated with increased heart disease risk.

The presence of a certain amino acid and proteins in the blood can indicate whether or not an individual is in a high risk category for heart disease. Elevated homocysteine levels (associated with a folic acid deficiency; see Chapter 7) are associated with a higher risk of heart disease and stroke. The presence of a protein called C-reactive protein in our blood also indicates an increased risk of heart disease. Research has shown that high levels of C-reactive protein, a marker of inflammation, increased the risk of heart disease by over four times [137]. Other useful markers are oxidative stress and lipoprotein (a) [138].

The cholesterol/statin controversy

Statins in herbal medicines

Statins were first isolated from the Chinese natural medicine red yeast rice, which has been used as a natural blood tonic for many centuries. Modern research has shown this remedy to have cholesterol-lowering properties, attributed to its component statins, the most abundant being lovastatin at 0.2% of the dry weight. The therapeutic dose contains some 4.5mg lovastatin which is five to ten times less than the standard recommended dose of synthetic lovastatin. This indicates that the medicine contains other components with beneficial properties such as plant sterols, isoflavones and monounsaturated fatty acids.

118

Several human clinical trials have been carried out with this medicine. Two eight-week studies indicated a reduction in total and LDL cholesterol with HDL levels either rising or remaining constant. Short-term side effects such as gastric upset, sleep disturbance, muscle pain (myalgia), fatigue, peripheral neuropathy and hepatotoxicty, commonly seen with high-dose synthetic statin treatments, were not observed in these studies. However, any unequivocal benefits of this natural medicine in the treatment of CVD have not been demonstrated.

Low dose statins may have beneficial effects

Recent research has suggested that low dose statins exert their mild positive effects by reducing inflammation and vascular calcification and not by reducing LDL cholesterol. This is very important information which supports the role of statins as therapeutic agents, and it is a great puzzle that the pharmaceutical industry and the great majority of the medical profession continue to pursue the cholesterol route which requires a much higher dose, has dubious benefits, and potentially dangerous side effects.

Metabolites affected by statin therapy

Cholesterol is not the only vital component in the body that is lowered by statin drugs. These drugs also inhibit the production of coenzyme Q10, which is crucially important in energy metabolism. Coenzyme Q10 levels always decrease naturally with age, so treatment with statins will have dangerous consequences in further depressing the energy levels of ageing patients, reducing their physical activity still further. Anecdotal evidence suggests that statin treatment can result in a lack of energy, muscle pain following moderate exercise and is associated with more frequent memory lapses. A recent study linking Parkinson's disease with low blood cholesterol challenges the wisdom of statin therapy. There are more than 200 messenger molecules called G-proteins, involved in the control of bodily functions, particularly of the brain, which have lipid side chains that enable them to anchor to cell membranes. These lipid molecules are formed on the same pathway as cholesterol and will also be affected by statin administration.

A great majority of the informed public must now be aware of the use of statins as a strategy for the lowering of LDL cholesterol for the treatment and prevention of heart disease. A closer investigation reveals that the role of LDL cholesterol as a risk factor in heart disease has not been proven, despite the expenditure of many millions of dollars. The Framingham Heart Study alone invested some 17 million dollars in an inconclusive long-term investigation. Despite a high mortality rate in an initial trial, statin drugs fuel a multibillion dollar industry. Prominent scientists and particularly high ranking medical researchers in heart disease have even suggested the universal use of statins to prevent heart disease in men over 50.

Press reports invariably quote uncritical views of the statin lobby who sing the praises of these drugs as the ultimate answer to heart disease. A more sober assessment is in order. Early trials did not bode well for heart patients when, according to press reports, the use of cerivastatin was linked to rhabdomyolysis, which led to kidney failure, and was responsible for 31 fatalities in the US and a further 21 deaths worldwide. In addition, 385 non-fatal cases were reported among the estimated 700,000 users of cerivastatin in the US, most of whom required hospitalisation. This resulted in the voluntary withdrawal of cerivastatin from the market.

Deregulation of statin use in the UK

A most alarming development in recent years has been the removal of the cholesterol-lowering statins from the prescribed drug category in the UK. Full page advertisements are appearing in colour magazines which exhort middle-aged women to have their cholesterol levels checked, not by doctors but by pharmacists who may recommend subsequent treatment with statins. Despite the expenditure of many millions of dollars and the publication of thousands of scientific papers, there is still no clear consensus on what constitutes a healthy level of cholesterol. There needs to be a major re-evaluation of the role of cholesterol in general health.

Over the past three decades, a large body of evidence has been accumulated which demonstrates that these drugs can have extremely dangerous and life-threatening consequences. It is exceptionally puzzling to us why these drugs have escaped the normally scrupulous assessment of the regulatory authorities who have banned many less toxic drugs. A full exposé of the efficacy and risks of statin treatment would require a separate and extensive book. This section is a brief attempt to counter the many unrealistic claims made for the benefits of statin therapy.

The biochemical effects of statins

Statins inhibit a crucial enzyme which controls many biosynthetic pathways in cells and tissues. This enzyme, HMGCoA-reductase for short, catalyses the formation of mevalonic acid, a precursor for vital cell membrane components such as cholesterol, Coenzyme Q (a respiratory electron carrier) and many G-proteins (over 200 at the latest count) with vital roles in cell metabolism, division and differentiation. Cholesterol and G-protein depletion have been implicated in several neurodegenerative conditions,

121

including Parkinson's disease. Low blood cholesterol has been linked to neurological dysfunction associated with depression, aggression, suicidal tendencies and memory loss.

All human cells contain cholesterol in their membranes but nerve cells in particular require an optimum cholesterol content to maintain healthy electrical conductance in neurotransmission. This may explain the occurrence of neurological dysfunction in some people with low cholesterol.

Low blood cholesterol is also associated with an increased risk of haemorrhagic stroke. In the latter half of the past century cholesterol levels in the 'healthy' Japanese population were relatively low (average 4.0mM) compared with a US or UK average closer to 6.0. Whilst the incidence of CVD was much lower in Japan, the incidence of haemorrhagic stroke was slightly higher than in the US. As the Japanese diet became more westernised, the average blood cholesterol level rose and the incidence of haemorrhagic stroke fell close to Western values. However, the higher cholesterol levels did not result in any increase in CVD incidence, thus questioning the wisdom of using statins to combat heart disease by lowering blood cholesterol.

Coenzyme Q (ubiquinone)

Ubiquinone is found in all aerobic cells in the mitochondrial membranes, where it plays an essential part in the release of energy in aerobic respiration. The highest concentrations of ubiquinone are found in heart muscle where 40% of the weight is composed of mitochondria. As we age, we produce less ubiquinone and we are therefore less able to perform endurance or power exercises. Any further reduction in the production of ubiquinone will further reduce our ability to exercise.

Statins can interfere with energy metabolism and muscle performance by several different mechanisms:

1. Energy for muscle contraction is provided by both aerobic and anaerobic production of ATP, the fuel for muscle contraction. Statins can inhibit both these processes.

   a) Aerobic respiration requires coenzyme Q10 (ubiquinone) which is formed from mevalonate which is depleted by statin administration.

   b) The anaerobic respiration of glucose units by glycolysis is stimulated by the stress hormone adrenaline, which acts via G-proteins to accelerate muscle glycogen breakdown during high intensity activity. Statins inhibit the synthesis of all G-proteins.

2. The control of muscular activity by nerve impulses can also be affected by the statin mediated inhibition of mevalonate production.

3. If cholesterol levels fall below 3.0mM, nerve fibre membranes can become depleted of cholesterol, leading to loss of insulating function and neurotransmission.

4. The growth, maintenance and differentiation of nerve cells also requires the action of G-proteins and this in turn will control the response of muscle cells to nervous and chemical stimuli.

5. Calcium ions are absolutely essential for the process of muscle contraction, and their concentration in the muscle cell is controlled by a complex pathway called the 'phosphoinositide cascade'. This pathway is mediated by G-proteins. In addition to opening calcium channels in

123

cell membranes, this cascade also activates the enzyme protein kinase C. This multifunctional enzyme plays a crucial role in cell division and proliferation, involved in muscle growth and regeneration.

Statins and muscle function

The commonest manifestation of statin side effects is seen in muscle tissue, as a result of the inhibition of coenzyme Q synthesis. This inhibits the function of the highly aerobic Type 1, coenzyme Q-dependent muscle fibres which normally function in all low intensity exercise. The body responds by switching to the Type 2b fibres which normally function in high intensity exercise and do not require oxygen and coenzyme Q. This leads to a build-up of lactate that would not normally occur if the Type 1 muscle fibres were fully active. This is most probably responsible for the fatigue and muscle pain reported in up to 20% of statin users.

This may also account for the wealth of anecdotal evidence, particularly from older statin users, of a lack of energy and disinclination to exercise. Popular health food magazines are now urging statin users to take coenzyme Q to overcome the unwanted side effects. The statin manufacturers used to include coenzyme Q in their original statin pills, as from the outset, they were well aware of the need to maintain this essential cofactor at an optimum concentration in the body. Coenzyme Q is not included in the latest statin formulations, presumably as a result of its high cost.

Statin myotoxicity follows a clear progression with increasingly severe symptoms.

1. Asymptomatic elevation of the enzyme creatine kinase which is a marker for the switch to anaerobic muscle metabolism.

2. Myalgia (muscle pains).

3. Muscle necrosis or breakdown.

4. Severe muscle degeneration or rhabdomyolysis which is invariably fatal.

Genetic susceptibility to statin treatment

The genetic basis for the role of ubiquinone in aerobic muscle function has been studied in man where mutations in the CO Q2 gene cause reductions in coenzyme Q biosynthesis and consequent defects in respiration and muscular efficiency. Patients with such genetic conditions will be particularly susceptible to the damaging effects of statins. In a recent pharmacogenetic study, all patients with the common mild genetic variation in the CO Q2 gene showed significant statin intolerance [139]. Other less common congenital disorders involving the mevalonate pathway in membrane glycosylation linked to diabetes, liver disease and increased blood clotting will be exacerbated by statin therapy with potentially fatal consequences.

Health risks associated with excessively low LDL cholesterol

Many doctors in the UK appear to be advising their patients to reduce their cholesterol levels to an 'optimum' of 3.0mM. This is extremely unwise for the following reasons. Even without statin treatment, low blood cholesterol has been associated with:

- Haemorrhagic stroke
- Depression

- Increased suicide risk

- Polyneuropathy: irreversible nerve damage with loss of sensory and motor functions.

- High risk of cancer mortality, especially in hyper-responders to statins, i.e. those where the drop in LDL cholesterol is very rapid.

- Increased mortality in patients with heart failure

- Parkinson's disease.

Since statins were developed primarily to lower LDL cholesterol then it follows that they will contribute to the above conditions in susceptible patients.

Statins and birth defects

A cause of grave concern is the potential effect on foetal development. Cellular growth and development in the foetus requires a rich supply of LDL cholesterol from the maternal blood. If the mother is on statins, then the cholesterol level may fall below the optimum for healthy foetal growth. There is some evidence that statins can cause severe birth defects if the mother has been taking statins in the first trimester of the pregnancy. Doctors advise women of child-bearing age against statin therapy, but there is a risk in the UK where statins can be bought without a prescription, that the woman then becomes pregnant and may not see a doctor for several weeks.

Effects of dietary components and other drugs on statin activity

Statins and all other drugs have to be eliminated from the body in order to prevent unwanted side effects. This complex process is carried out, mainly in the liver, where organic compounds are detoxified by a wide range of enzymes prior to excretion via the kidneys into the urine. For example, one particular enzyme Cytochrome P_{450} 3A4 is responsible for the clearance of several statins and other drugs shown in Table 8.

Enzymes are rather like turnstiles at a football game which allow only one person through at a time. Competition for the active site (turnstile) of the enzyme by several different molecules will slow down the metabolism of individual compounds. Note in Table 8 that statins and warfarin are cleared by the same enzyme. Since heart patients may be on simultaneous treatment with statins and warfarin, it is essential that responsible physicians are aware of the implications. The activity of these enzymes control the persistence, concentration and activity of statins in the blood. If the drug is rapidly metabolised and cleared, then its effect will be minimised. This may lead the doctor to prescribe a higher dose which in turn can increase the perceived therapeutic and pathological effects. Conversely, if the statin is poorly metabolised, then its concentration in the blood remains high and sustained and perhaps allows for a more moderate dosage regime. Co-administration of other drugs such as warfarin will compete with the statins and lower their rates of

Table 8 **Drugs detoxified by Cytochrome P_{450} 3A4**

Statins	Other drugs
Atorvastatin	Cyclosporin A
Cerivastatin (now banned)	Lidocaine
Simvastatin	Quinidine
	(R)-Warfarin

clearance. The reverse is also true and statins will interfere with the clearance of other drugs.

Potential effects of normal dietary components on statin clearance

Our food contains a multitude of compounds which are cleared by the cytochrome enzymes. For example, the consumption of modest amounts of grapefruit juice (200ml) taken with 40mg/day of simvastatin was found to increase the plasma concentration of the statin by some 3.6 times. Thus grapefruit juice may increase the cholesterol lowering effect, but also the adverse effects of simvastatin [140]. This might be a concern for obese heart patients on statin and warfarin, if without consulting a doctor, they embark on a grapefruit-rich diet, as part of a calorie-controlled weight loss programme.

Having discussed the basic biochemical effects of statins in the section above, we would urge extreme caution in the use of high-dose statin therapy to reduce blood cholesterol levels as a strategy for CVD prevention and cure. The use of low-dose statin treatment to treat CVD via the anti-inflammatory effects of statins is acknowledged, but the level of research into the toxicology of statins is currently inadequate.

7   Other dietary essentials

In addition to protein, fat and carbohydrate, the body has
an absolute requirement for water, minerals, vitamins
and fibre, with nutraceuticals as non-essential but
beneficial components. This chapter explains the
biochemical roles of vitamins and nutraceuticals and
briefly discusses the other components.

Definitions

A nutrient can be defined as a component of food that is required
for normal growth and development, the lack of which causes
organ system or cell dysfunction that can be reversed upon
prompt re-introduction of the nutrient into the diet. Dietary
components that are required only in very small amounts are
termed micronutrients. All vitamins and most minerals are in this
category. Nutraceuticals are a separate class of micronutrients
that are not essential dietary components, but which confer
important health benefits.

Vitamins

Vitamins regulate biochemical reactions. They are 'helpers' in
many cell functions, and they are essential in the processes by
which other nutrients are digested and used by the body.
Vitamins cannot yield energy, but they are vital in helping the
body to release energy.

There are two classes of vitamins, fat-soluble and water-
soluble. The fat-soluble vitamins A, D, E, and K are carried

through the body in the LDL/HDL fat transport system. These vitamins are stored in body fat and the liver, and there may be a risk of toxic build-up if they are taken to excess. All other vitamins are water-soluble, so any excess is simply carried away in the urine. However, some vitamins can be dangerous if taken in large quantities or in combination with prescription drugs.

Most of us may have taken vitamin supplements, because we have read something somewhere about the health giving properties of particular vitamins, and have been confused by the jargon on the label of many vitamin supplements such as one capsule or tablet contains 100% RDA and/or X number of IU. The RDA or Recommended Daily (or Dietary) Allowance is an actual weight of material, usually measured in mg, whereas the IU or International Unit is a measure of the biological activity of the compound. For example, the RDA for vitamin E is 20mg which is equivalent to 29 IU, making 1mg of vitamin E equivalent to 1.45 IU.

In the absence of adequate dietary vitamins, dietary changes or supplementation may be required. In the developing countries, it has been estimated that up to 500,000 people every year become blind as a result of clinical vitamin A deficiency. This has been a moving force in the development of 'golden rice', a genetically engineered product enriched with vitamin A.

Sources of vitamins

Vitamins are best obtained from a healthy, well balanced and varied diet. As the food is digested, the vitamins are slowly released and absorbed from the intestine in a well-controlled process over a long time period. When vitamin supplements are taken, the process of uptake is very different, as unless the product is a slow release formulation, the vitamins are taken up more rapidly, which may overload the system. If the vitamins are oil-soluble like vitamin D, then they may accumulate in the body fat with potentially toxic effects. Water-soluble vitamins on the other hand are rapidly excreted into the urine to maintain an optimum blood concentration. Anyone who has taken vitamin B tablets very soon produces bright yellow urine.

Vitamins A, C and E have been studied in recent years for their antioxidant properties. These vitamins help to protect the body against free radicals that can damage cells and potentially result in cancer, premature ageing, Alzheimer's disease, arthritis and heart disease.

Vitamin A

This vitamin is required for a healthy skin and is essential for night vision. It is an antioxidant and stimulates the immune system. It may play a role in both the prevention and treatment of cancer by its involvement in the following cellular processes.

Immune stimulant

Too little vitamin A brings about changes in cell membranes and alters the function of the cells that are involved in our immune response to infection [141]. Scientific study has suggested that vitamin A supplementation may enhance recovery from measles [142] and reduce respiratory infections in children.

Cell division

Billions of cells are dividing in our body every day. A deficiency of vitamin A may result in errors in this process of cell proliferation, and the cell division process may result in the development of cancer. It has been demonstrated that vitamin A can cause cancer cells grown in the laboratory to lose their cancerous properties, and to grow more slowly like healthy cells.

Cell to cell communication

Healthy cells communicate with each other and with damaged cells. This helps to maintain coordination of our cellular functions and prevents damaged cells from proliferating and eventually progressing to become cancer cells. Vitamin A aids in this communication process and a deficiency can lead to a distortion or break in communication, potentially leading to tumour development [143].

Beef liver is the richest animal source of vitamin A. As β-carotene is the precursor for vitamin A, all vegetables and fruits containing this carotenoid are a valuable source of vitamin A, particularly carrots and sweet potatoes.

The B vitamins

The vitamin B complex refers to all of the known essential water-soluble vitamins except for vitamin C. The B complex vitamins are a group of similarly structured compounds, which is why we refer to them as a 'complex'. 'Vitamin B' was originally thought to be a single nutrient found in extracts of rice, liver or yeast. These extracts were later found to contain several vitamins, which were given different numbers. This has led to the mistaken belief that these vitamins have a special relationship to each other. Unlike the vitamins in the E complex, the B vitamins are not structurally related, but are all water-soluble. This group of compounds includes thiamine, riboflavin, niacin, pantothenic acid, pyridoxene and cobalmines.

Thiamine (vitamin B1)

Vitamin B1 is required in the processing of carbohydrates, fat, and protein. Every cell in the body requires vitamin B1 as it plays a vital role in producing the energy that the body needs for general metabolism and for the nerve cells to function normally. Low intake of thiamine is associated with an increased risk of prostate cancer [144]. Thiamine is often added back to enrich bread, but is not added to pastry flour. As we age and/or consume alcohol on a regular basis, our thiamine levels tend to drop [145]. The best sources of vitamin B1 are be found in wheat germ, whole wheat, peas, beans, enriched flour, fish, peanuts and meat.

Riboflavin (vitamin B2)

Vitamin B2 is also mainly involved with generating the energy the body needs from food. However, vitamin B2 is also essential for the generation of the powerful cellular protective enzyme glutathione peroxidase, which destroys free radicals and may play a role in reducing the risk of developing many chronic diseases. Although vitamin B2 is usually added back to bread and cereals, elderly people, regular alcohol consumers and the economically less well-off tend to have low vitamin B2 levels [146]. The best sources of vitamin B2 are dairy products and eggs. Meat contains significant amounts of vitamin B2, as do leafy green vegetables, whole grains, and enriched cereals and bread.

Niacin (vitamin B3)

As with vitamins B1 and B2, vitamin B3 plays a role in energy production from carbohydrates in the body. However, niacin has other functions which may help in the treatment of cancer patients. In animal tests, niacin supplementation was shown to reduce the damage to healthy cells caused by anti-cancer drugs such as adriamycin, but did not interfere with the tumour killing capacity of the drug [147]. Similarly, niacin appears to increase the efficiency of tumour cell killing in radiation therapy. Niacin can also act upon tumour cells to change the coating of the tumour; this makes it more susceptible to the body's immune system, as well as to medical intervention.

Niacin has been used as a cholesterol lowering treatment. Niacin lowers total cholesterol and LDL cholesterol yet raises the level of the 'good' HDL cholesterol [148]. However, relatively large doses of niacin are needed to have the desired effect of lowering blood cholesterol. If niacin is used for the purpose of lowering cholesterol care should be taken, as undesirable side effects such as skin flushing, stomach irritation, nausea, glucose intolerance, elevated blood levels of uric acid, visual disturbances and liver damage have been reported. In recent years a niacin derivative (niacin inosinate) has been used at high dosage with some success in lowering 'bad' cholesterol without any unpleasant side effects. Good sources of niacin are meat, fish, mushrooms and whole wheat.

Pantothenic acid (vitamin B5)

Vitamin B5 plays an essential role in energy production and is needed to make the vital neurotransmitter acetylcholine which allows nerve impulses to be conducted efficiently. It is also essential in producing, transporting, and releasing energy from dietary fats. Vitamin B5 is also involved in cholesterol synthesis and needed to manufacture vitamin D and steroid hormones.

Pantethine, a by-product of vitamin B5, has been reported to lower blood levels of cholesterol and TGs with no toxicity or side effects [148]. Lower cholesterol and TGs may provide protection from heart disease. Vitamin B5 also moderates the

134

stress response, balancing the adrenal hormones and manufacture of red blood cells. The best sources of vitamin B5 are liver, kidneys, yeast, and salmon, but most other foods, including broccoli, egg yolk and grains, contain some vitamin B5.

Pyridoxine (vitamin B6)

Vitamin B6 is essential in processing amino acids, the building blocks of all proteins and some hormones. Vitamin B6 helps to make serotonin and melatonin. Melatonin is a natural hormone that regulates the human biological clock and research has shown that melatonin induces sleep [150]. Vitamin B6 can also aid in the formation of several neurotransmitters and is therefore an essential nutrient in the regulation of our mental processes.

In combination with folic acid and vitamin B12, vitamin B6 lowers homocysteine levels, an amino acid linked to heart disease and stroke, and possibly other diseases as well, such as osteoporosis and Alzheimer's disease [151, 152]. Levels of vitamin B6 above normal may have a number of potential benefits for cancer patients:

1. Immune stimulation: may allow the immune system to recognise and act against a tumour [153].

2. Control of blood sugar: controlling blood sugar levels is vital in the fight against cancer [154]. Cancer cells have an absolute requirement for glucose as an energy source. Restricting glucose may control the tumour and allow the immune system to destroy cancer cells.

3. Protection of healthy cells from radiotherapy-induced damage [155].

4. May specifically inhibit growth of melanoma [156].

135

All of the above properties may play a role, along with traditional cancer treatments, in reducing the tumour burden and increasing survival rates of cancer patients. Good sources of vitamin B6 are raisins, cereal bran, lentils, liver, turkey and tuna.

Cobalamins (vitamin B12)

Vitamin B12 is vital for normal nerve cell activity and replication of DNA. Vitamin B12 also acts with folic acid and vitamin B6 to control homocysteine levels. Vitamin B12 deficiency causes fatigue. Studies have shown that even people with chronic fatigue who are *not* deficient in this vitamin may have increased energy levels after vitamin B12 injections, compared with control injections [157]. In a preliminary trial, 2,500–5,000 micrograms (μg) of vitamin B12, given by injection every two to three days, led to improvement in 50–80% of a group with chronic fatigue syndrome, with the most improvement appearing after several weeks of injections [158]. Oral B12 supplements are unlikely to obtain the same results as injectable B12, as the body's ability to absorb adequate amounts of B12 is relatively poor. The best sources are oysters, sardines, tuna, eggs and cheese.

Vitamin C

Vitamin C is essential for human health and unlike most other creatures we are unable to make our own vitamin C. Our requirement for this vitamin is seen as far back as the middle ages. During the age of exploration by sea, as many as half of the crew members of these expeditions would die of scurvy, as a result of leakage of blood into the tissues from fragile blood vessels. Eventually it was discovered by Captain Cook that limes could prevent and reverse scurvy. English ships were then required to carry limes on board for the prevention of scurvy, hence the English sailors were nicknamed 'Limies'. Indeed, vitamin C is also known as ascorbic acid, which literally means 'without scurvy'.

The multiple benefits of vitamin C

Vitamin C protects our body in many ways, not just from scurvy:

- It may help prevent or reduce allergic responses by lowering histamine release. Histamine is the compound released by our body that induces an allergic response and often causes reddening of the skin [159];

- It helps in bone formation. Vitamin C is required for the synthesis of collagen, the body's most abundant protein. Bones are formed and maintained via a collagen 'framework'. Vitamin C has been shown to be important in bone formation in children [160] but does not play a role by controlling bone mineral content, absorption or alkaline phosphatase activity [161, 162];

- Vitamin C also stimulates the activity of an enzyme called alkaline phosphatase. This enzyme releases phosphate form body stores for bone formation;

- Stimulation of the immune response. Vitamin C can enhance the body's resistance to an assortment of diseases, including infectious disorders and many types of cancer. It strengthens and protects the immune system by stimulating the activity of antibodies and immune system cells such as phagocytes and neutrophils [163].

- High blood sugar depresses the immune system by competing with vitamin C for uptake into white blood

137

cells. The white blood cells are the cells that engulf harmful bacteria and are needed for a strong immune system. They require a high internal concentration of vitamin C to protect them against the free radicals which they produce to destroy the ingested bacteria.

- High vitamin C therapy against cancer may work by limiting glucose uptake into the tumour cells, because both glucose and vitamin C compete for the same method of entry into the cell.

- Vitamin C acts as a powerful antioxidant [164] and free radical scavenger.

- It acts together with insulin to maintain a healthy blood sugar level [165, 166].

- It has a small but important role in the clearance of cholesterol [167].

- Vitamin C has a protective effect against heart disease by reducing the oxidation of LDL [168] to 7-oxocholesterol and by playing a role in inhibiting platelet aggregation and formation of fat deposits in our arteries [169].

- A major role of vitamin C in cancer prevention may be in the inhibition or prevention of cancer cells from breaking down connective tissue collagen, the protein that holds the body tissues in place. This prevents the metastatic spread of cancer to other sites of our body. Vitamin C also stimulates the collagen formation necessary for 'walling off' tumours and may prevent their spread [170].

- Vitamin C can protect against a number of chronic diseases. Population studies indicate that individuals with high intakes of vitamin C have a lower risk of a number of chronic diseases, including heart disease, cancer, eye diseases, and neurodegenerative conditions [171].

• Vitamin C plays a significant role in protecting against heart disease. Ageing populations are generally at risk of poor nutrition, often resulting in a fall in plasma vitamin C concentrations. A recent study has indicated that a low blood vitamin C concentration in the older British population is strongly predictive of cardiovascular disease mortality [172]. In addition, recent evidence suggests that individuals with a high serum vitamin C concentration have a significantly reduced risk of stroke [173].

Indeed, Linus Pauling, the winner of two Nobel prizes for science, suggested that cardiovascular disease is caused by a lack of vitamin C. His hypothesis states that a low level of circulating vitamin C leads to leakage of blood from veins and arteries. This can be caused by loosening of the connective tissue around blood vessels, causing cracks to appear and the loss of barrier function of the blood vessels themselves. This is what happens in scurvy. To counteract this blood leakage during chronic low vitamin C concentration, fat deposits in the artery wall at the area of the leakage to plug the gap and prevent blood loss. Although both natural protective phenomena, fatty deposits and the stiffening or calcification of arteries are the clinical symptoms of cardiovascular disease. This process is what may have protected our cavemen ancestors during long winters on vitamin C-poor diets. Vitamin C may play a significant role in preventing and actually reversing this fatty deposit formation. However our ancestors were probably not at risk of developing heart disease, since they did not consume large amounts of trans fatty acids, omega-6 fats and refined carbohydrates, were highly active, and probably died long before the onset of age-related arterial degeneration.

Vitamin D

This vitamin has a major function in maintaining body calcium levels for the building of strong and healthy bones. Vitamin D is essential in the diet if we are not exposed to sunlight. We make vitamin D in the body by the action of sunlight upon the skin. The sunlight converts cholesterol in the skin to vitamin D.

Modern studies of surviving Stone Age cultures indicate that our early ancestors obtained up to five times more vitamin D than we do today. This is probably because they tended to eat whole and not processed foods, large amounts of oily fish and they also tended to live outside in the sunshine. So, what are the health benefits of vitamin D?

- Regulation of calcium transport in and out of cells. This controls the process known as cell differentiation which has been shown to play a role in the development of cancer [174].

- Vitamin D inhibits the growth of breast cancer cells grown in culture (outside the body) [175] and may reduce the growth of human breast cancer cells [176].

- Vitamin D also inhibits of the growth of human prostate cancer cells by inducing the cells to enter a permanent non growing state [177].

Since vitamin D is consumed in the diet and produced in the skin if we are exposed to sunshine, is toxicity a problem? Dark skinned people in sunny climates have skin full of melanin, and this reduces the production of vitamin D in their skin. For dietary vitamin D to become a problem it has to be activated by the kidneys and liver, and both of these routes can act as safeguards against toxicity except in cases of extreme overdose.

One of the consequences of vitamin D deficiency, rickets, was prevalent among the poorer sections of some Asian communities in northern industrial towns in the UK in the 1950s, before the clean air legislation came into force. The air pollution was so extreme that insufficient sunlight penetrated to allow the conversion of cholesterol in their skin to vitamin D. It has been calculated that sufficient vitamin D can be synthesised in the cheeks of a fair-skinned child playing outside on a sunny winter's day. Conversely, high doses of vitamin D can be toxic, and have been the cause of death among early Arctic explorers who ate polar bear liver, a very rich source of vitamin D. There is also recent evidence that excess vitamin D, in the absence of adequate vitamin K_2, can stimulate calcification or hardening of the arteries, which is an independent risk factor for CVD.

The E vitamins

Vitamin E is a fat-soluble vitamin complex which contains eight closely related compounds with powerful antioxidant activity [178]. α-Tocopherol has been reported to be the most active or usable form of vitamin E for human health. The validity of this claim is now justifiably questioned. α-Tocopherol was originally described as a compound that maintained fertility in rats [179]. In fertility restoration tests, α-tocopherol is only 10% more effective than γ-tocopherol and 54% more active than β-tocopherol. However, there is no reason to suggest that tocopherol used as a fertility agent will correlate with other biological activity such as antioxidant potential.

Antioxidants such as vitamin E act to protect our cells by scavenging free radicals (see Appendix). Free radicals can cause damage to our cells that may contribute to the development of cardiovascular disease, diabetes and cancer.

141

Unlike many other vitamins, the synthetic vitamin E or α-tocopherol is only one of the eight tocopherols found in the natural mixture, and it is not as active as the vitamin E complex. This suggests that we are much better off getting our vitamin E from natural food sources rather than from a supplement.

Which foods provide vitamin E?

Nuts, wheat germ, green leafy vegetables and oily fish are the main dietary sources of vitamin E. Fortified cereals are also an important source of vitamin E. Vegetable oils are not a recommended source with their high concentration of omega-6 fat. The RDA for vitamin E is 20mg or 29 IU. However, living in a polluted environment, and being exposed to pollution both from the air and the food we eat, we should probably take much more, possibly ten times this amount.

Can we suffer from vitamin E deficiency?

Vitamin E deficiency is very rare. It may occur in individuals who cannot absorb dietary fat, or if people are consuming a very low fat diet for extended periods. This has been seen in premature, very low birth weight infants and in sufferers from a rare disorder of fat metabolism. Vitamin E deficiency is usually characterised by neurological problems, primarily as a result of poor nerve conduction.

Who may need extra vitamin E?

All of our cellular membranes contain polyunsaturated fats, which are more easily damaged by free radicals than saturated fats. In order to protect our membranes, it is essential that we take natural vitamin E. Anyone diagnosed with cystic fibrosis, individuals who have had part or all of their stomach removed, individuals with malabsorptive problems such as Crohn's disease with reduced fat absorbtion, and smokers may need supplemental vitamin E. It should be noted here that large dose supplements of natural vitamin E should not be taken in the absence of adequate dietary vitamin C. Vitamin C serves to regenerate the active and protective form of vitamin E (see Appendix).

Most studies to date have been carried out using the synthetic form of vitamin E which is α-tocopherol. There is remarkably little information on the efficacy of the different components in natural vitamin E. Nature is usually very efficient and the evolution of this vitamin as a mixture of eight related compounds would not have occurred if α-tocopherol was the only useful antioxidant.

Society is increasingly moving towards low fat diets, a move driven by advice from physicians and nutritionists and propaganda from the processed food industry. The average low fat diet provides only about 7–11mg per day of vitamin E [180]. The recommended dietary allowance of vitamin E at the current time is 20mg. So, by eating a low fat diet, we may actually be consuming approximately half of the recommended amount of vitamin E and may absorb even less.

Epidemiological studies with vitamin E

What role, if any does vitamin E play in protection from chronic diseases such as cancer, heart disease, diabetes and obesity? It is very difficult to give a definitive statement on the role of the E vitamins because most dietary studies use the synthetic α-tocopherol, and retrospective studies involved sources both from supplements and the diet.

Vitamin E (α-tocopherol) and heart disease

Since most clinical trials actually used α-tocopherol rather than the natural E vitamin complex, we will use the precise name for the pure compound. Studies suggest that α-tocopherol may help prevent or delay CHD. Oxidative modification (damage caused by free radicals) of LDL cholesterol will promote blockages in coronary arteries, leading to atherosclerosis and heart attacks. α-Tocopherol may limit the oxidation of LDL cholesterol [181, 182]. However, recent clinical trials suggest that long term oral vitamin C and α-tocopherol do not improve atherosclerosis or reduce LDL cholesterol oxidation in the body [183, 184].

α-Tocopherol may also help to prevent the formation of blood clots, which could lead to a heart attack. The results from the Nurses' Study, involving around 90,000 nurses, suggested that the incidence of heart disease was reduced by 30% to 40% in subjects with the highest intake of vitamin E from diet and supplements. The range of intakes from diet and supplements was 32–1,500mg, with an average intake of 139mg per day, which is much more than the recommended daily allowance [185].

The Heart Outcomes Prevention Evaluation (HOPE) Study followed almost 10,000 patients who were at a high risk for heart attack or stroke for 4.5 years [186]. In this study, subjects receiving 265mg of α-tocopherol per day did not experience significantly fewer cardiovascular events or hospitalisations for heart failure or chest pain, when compared to those who did not receive vitamin E supplements.

The results of the latter study suggested that it is unlikely that diets supplemented with α-tocopherol provide any protection against cardiovascular disease. Is this true? A factor that the researchers did not take into account was the dietary regime of the subjects other than vitamin E supplementation.

People with increased risk of cardiovascular disease and/ or stroke tend to be on low fat diets, usually on the instruction of a doctor or dietician. The average low fat diet provides only about 7–11mg a day of vitamin E (well below the RDA) [180]. In this case dietary supplementation of α-tocopherol may be ineffective, since most of the supplement may not be taken up into the subject's body, due to a low fat diet and the fact that supplements may not be the best way to get vitamin E into the blood.

> **Low fat diets may increase the incidence of heart disease by reducing the uptake of vitamin E and other oil-soluble antioxidants.**

Recent reports have suggested that the huge variations in vitamin E absorbtion are dependent upon the type of delivery. Results suggested that cereal fortified with vitamin E allowed a very high rate of absorption of the vitamin into the bloodstream. Pills taken separately with the same but unfortified cereal had variable effects. Taking vitamin E supplements alone may be largely useless. This coupled to the low vitamin E uptake in people on low fat diets may account for variable results of studies involving vitamin E supplementation, particularly when only α-tocopherol is used as the supplement.

Vitamin E and cancer

E vitamins are powerful antioxidants and can help protect against the damaging effects of free radicals, many of which may contribute to the development of chronic diseases such as cancer,

145

heart disease and diabetes. Vitamin E may also block the formation of nitrosamines. These are carcinogenic compounds that are produced in the stomach from nitrite meat preservatives consumed in the diet [187].

E vitamins may also protect against the development of cancers by enhancing the function of our immune system [188]. Many trials investigating a protective effect of vitamin E as α-tocopherol on heart disease, and the association of vitamin E with the incidence of cancer, have been inconclusive. Not all studies have proven so, as α-tocopherol has been shown to protect against cancer of the prostate and stomach, and there is support for a protective role against colon cancer [56, 88, 189–191]. However, recent studies have suggested no protective effect of α-tocopherol from colon cancer development [192]. Some evidence associates higher intake of α-tocopherol with a decreased incidence of premenopausal breast cancer. However, an examination of the effect of α-tocopherol on incidence of post-menopausal breast cancer did not associate a greater α-tocopherol intake with a reduced risk of developing breast cancer [193].

Vitamin E and cataracts

Cataracts are damage to the lens of the eye that will ultimately lead to clouding of the vision, and this damage is caused by oxidation of the lens proteins by free radicals. Studies have found that lens clarity, which is used to diagnose cataracts, was better in regular users of vitamin E supplements and in persons with higher blood levels of vitamin E. However, a recent study investigating the incidence and rate of progression of age-related cataracts suggested that α-tocopherol supplementation had no effect upon cataract formation [194]. Further, a study involving middle aged male smokers did not demonstrate any effect from

146

α-tocopherol supplements on the incidence of cataract formation [195]. Smoking is a major risk factor for developing cataracts. However, the caroteoid lutein which is found in the eye is associated with protection against cataracts. This is found in fruit and vegetables, in particular the avocado, in association with the eight natural forms of vitamin E.

Natural vitamin E may be used as a preventative to reduce the risk of development of many disease states. However, studies concerning vitamin E and cataract formation, such as those mentioned above, used subjects where damage may have already began to accumulate. These studies may actually be looking for vitamin E to be a curative rather that preventative agent, and the two outcomes differ considerably.

The history of vitamin E research appears to follow a consistent pattern where early studies related natural vitamin E consumption and blood levels of the natural E vitamins to various disease symptoms. Where several studies revealed beneficial effects, these were followed up with supplementation trials using synthetic α-tocopherol. The results were often inconclusive or negative. These latter results do not disqualify the E vitamins as beneficial dietary constituents, but suggest that future trials should use the natural mixture of E vitamins, rather than the synthetic α-tocopherol. The associated diet should also contain enough fat to ensure uptake of the fat-soluble vitamins.

Can we get too much α-tocopherol?

A recent review of the safety of α-tocopherol in the elderly indicated that taking α-tocopherol supplements for up to four months at doses of 530mg or 800 IU, which is 35 times the current RDA, had no significant effect on general health, body weight, levels of body proteins, lipid levels, liver or kidney function, thyroid hormones, amount or kinds of blood cells and bleeding time [196]. Longer term safety of α-tocopherol or natural vitamin E supplementation has not been tested.

Based on the above studies, an increased intake of natural vitamin E seems prudent, but as with most other nutrients, the best source is through eating a healthy diet rather than taking a dietary supplement.

Recent exciting developments in vitamin E research

Could γ-tocopherol be the most active form of vitamin E? With contradictory and confusing results such as these, at this time there seems limited evidence for recommending synthetic vitamin E supplements for the prevention of cancer and other chronic diseases. A growing body of evidence suggests that another form of vitamin E, γ-tocopherol, is a better protective agent against heart disease and certain cancers. Crucially, supplementation with α-tocopherol leads to a depletion of γ-tocopherol in our body [197]. We can now begin to see why many of these studies involving supplementation with α-tocopherol alone may have given conflicting results. Plants have, after all, evolved a complex cocktail of antioxidants to protect their germ tissues against oxidative damage, and the oil-soluble mixture of at least eight vitamin E isomers plays a crucial role. Why try to improve on billions of years of evolution by cutting out seven of the eight isomers and giving α-tocopherol in large doses?

Recent research is beginning to show the subtle interplay between the various isomers of vitamin E. For example, α-tocopherol and γ-tocopherol have different protective functions in the cell, but they also control each other's uptake and residence

148

time in the body. Natural as distinct from synthetic vitamin E is rich in γ-tocopherol.

New protective functions for the E vitamins

The E vitamins have an important role in gene expression and cell signalling. In the past 15 years it has become apparent that the E vitamins have extremely important 'non-antioxidant functions'. They act as regulators of gene expression controlling the activity of protein kinase C, but further control the process of inflammation by reducing the production of cyclooxygenase 2 and prostaglandins.

Much previous vitamin E research was limited to α-tocopherol and this may have been responsible for the negative results obtained in several major clinical trials. More attention is now being given to the other dietary tocopherols as potential inhibitors of degenerative diseases, including CVD, cancer, and age-related cataracts. Very recently, δ-tocopherol has been found to have cooperative effects with α-tocopherol. All this new information further supports the need to obtain adequate amounts of the natural E vitamins in the diet. Small amounts occur in nuts, seeds, some vegetable oils and most natural fat-containing foods. Richer dietary sources include the germ/bran from wheat, rice and oats. More concentrated sources for use as supplements include wheat germ oil, rice bran oil and vitamin E rich palm oil fractions. We suggest that these latter supplements would be best taken in a mixture with omega-3 oils, from flax or oily fish, in order to protect the oxygen-sensitive oils from spoilage as well as adding to their anti-inflammatory roles in the body. Both of these types of natural molecules have crucial multifunctional roles in protecting our vital tissues against inflammation and damage.

149

In the case of the E vitamins, it cannot be stressed too strongly that not only do they directly combat oxidative stress, but they also reduce the expression of genes that control the process of inflammation (see Appendix) [198].

The K vitamin group

Vitamin K_1: phylloquinone

Vitamin K_1 was discovered in 1929 by the Danish scientist Hendrik Dam, as a component of the blood coagulation system. It was named phylloquinone to indicate its isolation from green plants where it plays a pivotal role in photosynthesis. Later research revealed a family of other related K_2 vitamins or menaquinones involved in fermentation processes in the human gut, cheese manufacture and fermented soya bean products. The K vitamin group as a whole can act as co-factors in blood coagulation and bone metabolism.

Sources of K vitamins

Vitamin K_1 is found in all green vegetables, but is only poorly absorbed if they are eaten raw, boiled or steamed. This oil-soluble vitamin is released when leaves are cooked in oil at a high temperature for a short time as in stir frying, when the bioavailability rises from 5% to 15% of the total K_1 content. The dietary K_2 vitamins are found at low concentrations in liver, milk, meat and fish, at intermediate levels in egg yolk, butter and curd cheeses, and at higher levels in soft and hard cheeses such as Gouda and Edam. The richest sources of K_2 are fois gras (goose liver) and a specialist fermented soybean product called natto, which has been eaten in Japan for at least 1,000 years. Dietary sources of K_2 vitamins are shown in Table 9 with concentrations expressed as micrograms (µg) per 100g of food.

In the UK, an arbitrary RDA for vitamin K_2 is quoted as 75µg. In the US, current recommendations for vitamin K_2 intake varies between 90–120µg for young adults. It is difficult to see how these levels can be achieved without the consumption of the more exotic foods shown in Table 9.. In fact, current research indicates that most Western populations are deficient in vitamin K_2 and that this may account, in part, for the increased rates of osteoporosis, limb fracture and heart disease when compared to Japanese populations. Even within Japan there are large regional differences in the incidence of the above conditions and these are closely associated with the consumption vitamin K_2-containing fermented soybean foods.

The K vitamins also have a vital role in the mineralisation or incorporation of calcium in bone, and recently have been found to inhibit and even reverse the process of vascular calcification, or hardening of the arteries. Vitamin D is often referred to as the crucial vitamin in bone formation, but this is an

Table 9   **Vitamin K_2 concentrations in foods**

Food	Vitamin K_2 concentration (µg per 100g)
Liver, meat, milk and fish	0.5–5.0
Egg yolk, butter and curd cheese	15–25
Soft and hard cheeses	55–75
Goose liver	370
Natto (*Bacillus subtilis* fermented soybeans)	1100

over-simplification. Vitamin D stimulates the uptake of calcium from the intestine into the blood prior to its incorporation into bone which requires vitamin K. Recently there have been articles in the press claiming that the RDAs for vitamin D are far too low and should be increased some tenfold. The K vitamins are not even mentioned, even though research shows that patients deficient in vitamin K are at higher risk of CHD when given booster doses of vitamin D. The increased blood calcium is deposited in the artery walls in the absence of adequate vitamin K.

Beneficial effects of the dietary K_2 vitamins

- K_2 vitamins are more readily absorbed from the diet than vitamin K_1.

- Vitamin K_1 has a half-life in blood of some three hours, whereas the longer chain K_2 vitamins can persist for up to 100 hours.

- They can replace K_1 in the processes of blood coagulation and bone formation.

- They reverse arterial calcification in animals previously treated with warfarin to induce calcification.

- They improve the elasticity of blood vessel walls.

- They may promote brain function by decalcifying the blood vessels of the brain. This has potential in the treatment of Parkinson's and Alzheimer's diseases.

- They prevent bone loss in glucocorticoid-treated patients, and postmenopausal women. Simultaneous administration of vitamin D_3 further enhances this effect.

152

- The risk of CVD is reduced by reducing coronary artery calcification. Note that this effect was not demonstrated in studies with K_1.

- Both *in vivo* and *in vitro* studies have demonstrated the anti-cancer effects of the K_2 vitamins. A wide variety of cancer cell types are growth-suppressed or destroyed by K_2 vitamins. Several studies with leukaemic patients on MK-4 treatment yielded complete cytogenetic remission. A Japanese trial with liver cancer patients showed significant improvement in survival with doses of 45mg/day of oral K_2. This dose is almost 1,000 times the UK RDA and may explain why vitamin K_2 therapy is not more widespread in the US and Europe.

Warfarin therapy, often in conjunction with statins, is the treatment of choice for patients at high risk of heart disease from blood clotting. One of the unfortunate long-term side effects of this therapy is that warfarin stimulates the process of vascular calcification by inhibiting the activity of vitamin K. While the short-term benefits of warfarin therapy are obvious, it may increase the risk of CVD mortality in the long term. Perhaps other strategies such as dietary modification, avoiding the high omega-6 pro-inflammatory vegetable oils and supplementation with natural vitamin E and fish oils and not smoking might provide a better long-term strategy.

Biotin

Biotin acts as an essential coenzyme in the metabolism of protein, fats and carbohydrates. Biotin is also essential for the production of an enzyme in the liver that is involved in the breakdown of glucose. Good dietary sources of biotin include liver and kidney, oatmeal, egg yolk, soy, mushrooms, bananas, peanuts and brewer's yeast. Bacteria in the intestine also produce significant amounts of biotin, but evidence is conflicting as to whether biotin produced by intestinal bacteria is present at a location or is in a form that permits significant absorption by the body [199].

Folic acid or folate

Folic acid is a B vitamin needed for cell replication and growth. Folic acid helps the body form the building blocks of DNA and RNA, the body's genetic information. The body needs RNA to make proteins for use in all cells. Rapidly growing tissues, such as those of an unborn baby, and rapidly regenerating cells, like red blood cells and the cells of the immune system, have a high requirement for folic acid. Folic acid deficiency may result in a form of anaemia and is often found in patients with leukaemia.

Several birth defects or even cancer can arise from a low-folate diet when cells grow erratically and DNA damage occurs. The requirement for folic acid is doubled during pregnancy [200]. Deficiencies of folic acid during pregnancy are associated with low birth weight and an increased incidence of neural tube defects in infants resulting in spinal bifida [201]. Results have suggested that women who were at high risk of giving birth to babies with neural tube defects were able to lower their risk by 72% by taking folic acid supplements prior to and during pregnancy [202]. Women of childbearing age may be wise to supplement their diets with 400µg per day of folic acid. Such supplementation would protect against the formation of neural tube defects during the time between conception and when the pregnancy is discovered. If a woman waits until after pregnancy to begin taking folic acid supplements, the risk of birth defects may not be reduced.

In adults, folic acid is needed to keep levels of homocysteine, an amino acid by-product, from rising in the blood [203]. An excess of homocysteine in our blood is associated with an increased risk of heart disease and stroke and may play a role in other diseases such as osteoporosis and Alzheimer's disease [152]. A diet low in folic acid has been associated with a high incidence of pre-cancerous polyps in the colon, suggesting that folic acid may prevent the development of colon cancer [204]. In addition, studies have shown that reduced folic acid levels are associated with an increase in the incidence of cancer in ulcerative colitis patients [205].

Folic acid and vitamin B12 work together in a number of important reactions in the body, and a deficiency in one can often be masked by an excess of the other. In 1996 the FDA in the US proposed that all enriched flour, rice, pasta, cornmeal and other grain products contain 140µg of folic acid per 100g. Among people who do not take vitamin supplements, this amount of food fortification has been associated with increased folic acid levels in their blood and decreased blood levels of homocysteine. Nevertheless, to prevent neural tube defects fully [201], evidence is mounting that this level of folic acid fortification in food is inadequate.

Folate and cancer development

In preliminary studies, it was found that total folic acid intake was not associated with overall risk of breast cancer [206]. However, among women who consume at least one alcoholic beverage per day, the risk of breast cancer appears to be associated with a low folic acid intake. Moreover, multivitamin dietary supplements have also been associated with a lower breast cancer risk among women who consume at least 1.5 alcoholic beverages per day. Clearly, in the case of folic acid, dietary supplementation is recommended. The best dietary sources of folic acid are beans, leafy green vegetables, citrus fruits, beetroot, wheat germ and meat.

Nutraceuticals

These are organic compounds commonly found in plants and often referred to as phytonutrients. Like the vitamins they can be classified as oil-soluble or water-soluble.

Oil-soluble nutraceuticals

The most common nutraceuticals are the yellow, orange and red pigments found in vegetables and some fruit. They are termed carotenoids after β-carotene, which is responsible for the orange colour of carrots. Lycopene is a related red pigment found in tomatoes and some watermelons and grapefruit. Maize grains and avocado are a rich source of the yellow carotenoid, lutein, and red peppers contain capsanthin. Salmon flesh contains the orange carotenoid astaxanthin derived from the salmon's shellfish diet. All these carotenoids have potent antioxidant properties and can protect lipid membranes.

Carotenoid pigments

A dietary precursor of vitamin A, β-carotene is a compound known as a carotenoid. Carotenoids are found in nearly all yellow vegetables, particularly in carrots, and green vegetables. Carotenoids assist plants in the process of photosynthesis and also help to protect plants from the damaging effects of the sunlight and oxygen.

A large number of studies have shown that diets rich in fruit and vegetables will lower our risk of developing a range of chronic diseases including heart disease and cancers. Due to their presence in many fruit and vegetables, β-carotene and other carotenoids have been studied extensively as protective agents from chronic diseases. Dietary studies have suggested that carotenoids can affect the actions of many cancer causing agents in our bodies [207], possibly by maintaining normal cell to cell communication. This may help prevent or even reverse abnormal growth. However, carotenoids can affect the cancer process in a number of other ways.

Once the DNA in a cell in our body has been damaged, carotenoids may help to prevent the cell transforming into a cancer cell by stimulating cell to cell communication and re-differentiation [208]. Other work has suggested a role for β-carotene in enhancing cellular transformation, particularly in smokers and asbestosis sufferers [209], but not in healthy control patients. Carotenoids can protect our DNA against the damaging effects of many cancer causing agents [210].

Carotenoids have been shown to possess antioxidant activity [211]. Virtually no toxicity is associated with dietary carotenoids, except mild pigmentation of the skin following huge doses. Based on the positive evidence from dietary studies, supplementation programmes were instigated in the mid 1990s using pure or chemically synthesised carotenoids.

The National Cancer Institute initiated a study to determine whether β-carotene could reduce the incidence of lung cancer in heavy smokers. Results of this study suggested that it did not [212]. Further, two other studies indicated a substantial rise in the incidence of lung cancer in the β-carotene treatment group [213]. What did this mean? Were carotenoids actually causing, instead of protecting against cancer?

The authors of this book have performed studies indicating that carotenoids may protect cells at low or the normal concentrations circulating in the body. However, once this normal level is exceeded, the carotenoids lost their protective effect and may actually cause cellular damage themselves [214].

The point that needs to be made here is that nowhere in nature can be found a fruit or vegetable that contains only one form of carotenoid. Most if not all will contain a large number of different carotenoids in addition to a host of other protective agents that may all act in concert to confer protection. Isolation of one component from this mixture for further studies distorts the true picture of what that component can do for health. In addition, purified sources of carotenoids will be released into the body much more rapidly than from a natural food source, which is slowly and steadily released during digestion. The latter is an ideal situation, as the body needs a constant optimal concentration of nutrients and not sudden bursts provided by purified dietary supplements.

The pepper family are a particularly rich source of vitamin C when eaten raw and are a perfect accompaniment to a barbecue where they allow you to consume potentially toxic but delicious, chargrilled steaks which can be a source of dangerous free radicals. Vitamin C is a potent free radical scavenger which acts in concert with the pepper carotenoids. Furthermore, roasting the peppers makes the carotenoids more bioavailable, as in the case of tomatoes. Peppers and particularly hot chillies contain a powerful oil-soluble irritant called oil of capsicum or capsaicin. Anyone who has inadvertently wiped their eyes during the preparation of these peppers will have experienced the extreme burning sensation and will not repeat the mistake. This irritant oil has two useful applications. When applied to injured joints and muscles where the skin has not been damaged, it increases the blood supply and eases the pain, possibly by stimulating the body's natural pain suppressors, the endorphins. It is also thought to have anti-cancer properties by causing cancer cells to self-destruct, but overconsumption could lead to excessive irritation and may initiate cancer.

As far as studies concerning β-carotene supplementation for heavy smokers are concerned, after 30 years of smoking, the damage is already done. Dietary supplementation with high dose β-carotene alone will not prevent or reverse this damage. Indeed, as we have previously mentioned, β-carotene may enhance the damage. Diets rich in fruit and vegetables which will provide a combination of protective compounds including β-carotene and other carotenoids, released slowly during digestion, may significantly lower the incidence of cancer development in non-smokers. The following two examples demonstrate how one food source can supply several beneficial micronutrients, in addition to protein fat and carbohydrate.

The nutritional benefits of the tomato

Tomatoes contain carotenoids. Dietary studies have suggested that carotenoids such as β-carotene can affect the actions of many cancer-causing agents in our bodies [208], possibly by maintaining normal cell to cell communication.

Eating tomatoes, tomato ketchup, tomato sauce and pizza topped with tomato paste more than twice a week has been suggested to reduce the risk of prostate cancer by as much as 35%. Lycopene, the most abundant tomato derived carotenoid in blood serum and the compound that makes tomatoes red, was suggested to be the protective agent and was most efficiently absorbed into the blood in the presence of dietary fats [215]. Lycopene has been shown to inhibit tumours of the cervix [216], breast and lung in women [217]. Tomatoes are good for our eyes. Lycopene has been shown to act as a antioxidant that guards against age-related macular degeneration, a condition that may cause blindness [218]. Lycopene has also been shown to protect against heart disease by reducing the oxidation of LDL cholesterol [219]. In addition to containing lycopene and other carotenoids with potential protective effects, tomatoes are high in vitamin A, vitamin C, calcium, potassium and folate. Folate can protect against cancer and spina bifida. Potassium has been shown to produce a slight but definite drop in blood pressure [220, 221]. Current evidence suggests that dietary potassium may protect people who eat too much salt (see Appendix) [222].

The nutritional benefits of the avocado

Many people appreciate the delicious flavour of avocados, but avoid them because they believe they have a high fat content. Although avocados do contain fat, it is mostly the healthy monounsaturated kind, which has been shown to increase HDL and lower LDL, and they are themselves free of cholesterol. Avocados can provide us with many health benefits. They contain high quality essential fatty acids and proteins. Avocados are an excellent source of dietary fibre, particularly soluble fibre, which may promote faecal bulking and reduce faecal transit time, and have been suggested to lower risk of colon cancer development and lower blood cholesterol levels. They are a good source of several important amino acids, the antioxidant vitamin E and folate, which is required for the metabolism of DNA. Avocados are also a rich source of the carotenoid lutein which protects against macular degeneration.

Potassium is critical for nerve impulse transmission, muscle contraction, and as previously stated, heart function. Avocados provide more potassium than bananas and also provide a significant level of magnesium, a metal involved in carbohydrate and fat metabolism. In addition to being a highly nutritious food source, avocados can have marked advantages in skin care. Avocado oil is noted for a marked softening, soothing nature and its notable absorption when compared with almond, corn, olive and soybean oils [223]. Finally, avocados have been shown to contain an unusual sugar, mannoheptulose. This sugar has been shown to block glucose uptake by cells and may be a useful dietary means of controlling the growth and development of tumour cells which have an absolute requirement for glucose.

Foods containing water-soluble nutraceuticals

The brassicas

All of the brassicas or cabbage family, which includes broccoli, Brussels sprouts, cabbages and watercress, are highly beneficial to health. It has been thought since Roman times that diets rich in cabbage were protective against cancer and that cabbage leaves applied to wounds accelerated the healing process. More recently, studies in China have shown that cabbage-rich diets protect against stomach cancer. Current research has identified a class of water-soluble, pungently flavoured compounds called glucosinolates, found particularly in watercress and mustard. These compounds have been shown to be potent anti-cancer agents. One of their modes of action is to cause cancer cells to self destruct. Brassicas also have a protective function against heart disease by virtue of their rich content of antioxidant vitamins and pigments.

Onions and garlic

Onions and garlic contain volatile sulphur-containing compounds, which have anti-tumour activity and have been shown, along with the flavonoids and polyphenols, to lower blood pressure and blood lipids. Together with olive oil and tomatoes, garlic is a crucial component of the Mediterranean diet.

Water-soluble nutraceuticals found in fruit

Some of these micronutrients have already been mentioned in the preceding section on vegetables; however, it is fruit which provides a major supply of these compounds, in addition to minerals, vitamins and fibre.

Apples

Apples are a good source of vitamins and minerals. The skin contains water-soluble quercetin and several other antioxidant polyphenols with valuable anti-cancer and anti-heart disease properties. Apples are also a rich source of pectin, which aids water retention in the intestine and can help prevent constipation.

Apricots

Apricots are low in sugar, rich in potassium, and they contain both oil-soluble and water-soluble antioxidant pigments. The kernel is rich in an anti-cancer compound called laetrile, which is used in alternative medicine.

Bilberries

Bilberries and their American equivalent blueberries are a particularly rich dietary source of the powerful purple pigments, the antioxidant anthocyanins, which protect the retina in the eye from photooxidation caused by ultraviolet light. They also act synergistically with lutein from vegetables to further protect the visual process.

Cranberries

Cranberries contain beneficial antioxidants and in addition have antibacterial properties, particularly against infections of the bladder and urogenital tract.

Grapes

Components of the red grape are thought to be partly responsible for the French paradox where the consumption of red wine is associated with a decreased risk of heart disease. The protective components are thought to reside in the grape skin, as a complex mixture of polyphenols and flavonoids. One of the principal protectants appears to be resveratrol. These beneficial effects are lost when overconsumption of red wine can lead to alcohol-induced liver damage and ultimately cirrhosis.

Plums, strawberries and cherries

These fruits can be considered together as a good source of minerals, hydrophilic fibre (which aids the digestive process) and water-soluble antioxidant pigments.

Food quality

Chilled foods

Many people believe that chilled foods are as healthy as fresh produce, and sales of chilled foods are increasing rapidly in Europe and the US. Prepared chilled foods such as chopped salad with mayonnaise should be treated with caution because of the risk of bacterial contamination and possible food poisoning with salmonella and *E. coli*. Chilling is presumed to prevent the growth of these organisms, which grow best at body temperature (37°C). However, it has been demonstrated that these pathogens can survive and even grow slowly at lower temperatures.

Modified atmosphere packaging

This is another invention of the food industry to prolong the shelf life of salad vegetables. You may have noticed that a cut fresh lettuce placed in the fridge will have brown areas on the cut surfaces in the morning. This is unsightly but not harmful and is due to a natural oxidative process. To prevent this, salad vegetables are packaged in a low oxygen atmosphere in plastic bags (containing carbon dioxide or nitrogen) and may have a shelf life of up to two weeks. By this time there is a large loss in nutrient value and antioxidant vitamin content in apparently fresh-looking vegetables. These products are often labelled as being packaged in a protective atmosphere to reassure the public. If fresh vegetables are not readily available, one should always choose frozen vegetables over canned. The only worthwhile exceptions to this rule are tinned tomatoes and puree which are a valuable source of the carotenoids lycopene and β-carotene.

Other dietary essentials

Water, minerals and fibre

A discussion on diet would not be complete without reference to water, minerals and fibre. However, a comprehensive review is not appropriate since a consensus view has now been established on the optimum intake of minerals and dietary fibre, and can be found in a wide variety of advisory texts. Although not strictly a nutrient, water is essential for survival and good health. Indeed, we can survive no more than seven days without water, but a 40-day fast with water, minerals and vitamins is well within the capabilities of a healthy adult. Establishing a clean source of drinking water is crucial for good health and adequate water consumption has the following benefits:

- Excess water consumed has to be removed via the kidneys and this requires energy, which can be a valuable aid to weight loss. Conversely even mild dehydration can reduce the metabolic rate cause weight gain.

- Even one glass of water taken before bedtime can reduce night hunger pangs and midnight snacking.

- The average person should drink at least two pints of water per day and this should be increased with increasing physical activity.

Consumption of caffeine and alcohol-containing drinks should not replace water as these compounds are diuretic. Recent research indicates that the consumption of five to ten glasses of water per day can substantially reduce back and joint pain and the risk of cancers of the colon, bladder and breast.

Water: the essential nutrient

Essential for nearly all physiological functions, water helps to maintain body temperature, to lubricate and cushion our organs and joints, transport nutrients, and flush toxins from our body. The body needs water, even when we do not feel thirsty. Everyone should drink at least two pints of water per day, and an active person should drink much more. Any beverage can fulfil the requirement, except alcohol and caffeine-containing drinks, which are diuretics, but water is the healthiest and the most thirst-quenching. The human body contains between 55–75% water depending upon the ratio of body fat to muscle and it plays a vital role in every function of the body. As a rough guide, the following percentages can be applied:

Organ	% Water
Human brain	75%
Blood	92%
Muscles	75 %
Bones	22%

A glance at the above points should indicate that dehydration is not good for health. Even a mild state of dehydration will slow down our metabolic rate down by as much as 3%, and thus may play a role in weight gain. Furthermore, every drop of water consumed involves calories being used as the kidneys remove the excess water from our bodies. This is a valuable and painless aid to weight loss. Coupled with the findings that one glass of water prevented midnight feelings of hunger for almost 100% of individuals tested and the implications for weight control are obvious. Some 75% of Americans may be chronically dehydrated, and this fact likely applies to half of the world's population.

Preliminary research has indicated that 8–10 glasses of water a day could significantly ease back and joint pain for up to 80% of sufferers. Drinking five glasses of water daily has been suggested to decreases our risk of colon cancer development by 92% [224]. The same regular consumption of water has been suggested to cut the risk of bladder cancer by 49% [225] and of breast cancer development by a staggering 79%, although the data are sparse and inconsistent for breast cancer, but trying this strategy could help and will certainly not do any harm.

Drinking water quality

Drinking water quality deserves special consideration. The recommendation to drink only bottled water may not solve the problem. In the 1990s, New York's piped water supply was found to be of a higher quality than several bottled waters. There was also the case of a certain French product found to be contaminated with the carcinogen benzene. The water in our coffee or tea, or that which we use to reconstitute our orange juice or infant formula, may contain some atoms of lead from the pipes in our home or a minute amount of pesticide from a farm upstream. When necessary, bottled water can be a good temporary solution. Unfortunately, bottled water is regulated no more strictly than tap water, and enforcement is minimal, so there is no assurance that bottled water is safer to drink than tap water. Check with any water supplier, public or private, to assess the water purity.

Home water filters can be another good temporary solution if your tap water is unsafe. You must be sure the filtration capabilities of your filter match the contaminants in your water. Some filters improve the taste and odour of water while doing nothing to remove microbes or toxins. Home filtration of drinking and cooking water is the most cost effective and safe solution, but the filter characteristics and performance must be carefully checked, paying particular attention to the filter life. A good filter must remove both heavy metals and organic pollutants and last at least six months before requiring replacement.

The above is by no means a complete list of the potential hazards associated with drinking tap water. We feel that an extensive review of water contamination is beyond the scope of this text. However, the establishment of a healthy drinking water supply should be the first priority in any programme of dietary improvement, and the reader should not be put off drinking water by the above reports.

Minerals

Minerals, like vitamins, are essential for health. They help to build bones, the blood to carry oxygen, maintain cellular integrity, aid in energy production and muscle contraction and carry nerve signals all over the body. The correct mineral balance is important as minerals will compete for absorption in the intestine, so excess amounts of one mineral can actually inhibit absorption of others.

Fourteen different minerals have been shown to be essential to our health. These are: calcium, chromium, copper, fluorine, iodine, iron, magnesium, manganese, molybdenum, phosphorus, potassium, selenium, sodium and zinc.

Minerals that we require in relatively large amounts are called macro minerals. Those minerals that we need in small quantities are called micro minerals or trace minerals. We get these essential minerals primarily through the foods we eat. Good sources of essential minerals include fruits, vegetables, meats, nuts, beans and dairy products. Adequate amounts of minerals will be obtained from most normal diets. Supplementation is generally not necessary.

Fibre

Fibre is a term describing the substances in plant food which are not digested. Fibre provides almost no calories. This group of compounds consists mainly of complex carbohydrates.

Although not digested in the small intestine, some of the soluble fibre will be metabolised by our own bacteria in the large intestine. The resulting substances help acidify the colonic contents, resulting in water retention and faecal bulking. The faecal bulking and water retention by the stool enable a relatively rapid transit time for the stool. This may help protect the cells of the large intestine from the effects of ingested toxins and the harmful effects of bile acids and faecal water, potentially reducing our risk of developing colon cancer [226].

In addition, fibre consumption has recently been associated with a reduction in weight gain and insulin levels. Dietary fibre can also help to reduce the risk of developing heart disease and has been shown to play a role in reducing blood pressure. Dietary fibre has also been shown to play a role in reducing the level of LDL cholesterol and TGs, both risk factors for heart disease [227].

8   Beyond diet: exercise and stress

This chapter considers how exercise and stress are involved in the prevention of disease and the maintenance of good health. Exercise regimes are suggested for those suffering from obesity, diabetes, heart disease and cancer, and scientific evidence is presented for the role of exercise in the prevention of these diseases. The important role of stress in the progression of these diseases is also discussed.

Introduction

Before examining the crucial role of exercise in lifestyle improvement we briefly return to diet, because without sensible dietary changes, the benefits of exercise cannot be fully achieved. All the strategies discussed here involve the maintenance of or an increase in muscle mass, with improvements in blood parameters (optimised insulin, glucose and lipids), and body fat loss in the case of the obese. A large body of sound scientific evidence now points to the superior effects of low carbohydrate/high fat and protein diets in conjunction with exercise programmes for the treatment of many diseases and metabolic defects [228].

For our earliest ancestors, taking regular exercise was not much of an issue. Everyday survival itself involved physically demanding tasks, such as the gathering of food, hunting and fighting, and often required travelling great distances. More recently, particularly since the industrial revolution, the food that we consume and the way that we live has drastically changed. We

171

no longer use large amounts of energy gathering food to eat. With very little effort, we can gain access to an abundance of many different foods. We do use some energy working, but working for a living generally no longer involves heavy physical labour.

Regular physical activity is undoubtedly an essential part of good health and should be practised by everyone [190, 229]. Regular physical activity, not just as a guilt reflex after Christmas, will lower the risk of developing a number of chronic diseases including obesity, heart disease and cancer. For cancer survivors, the results of many studies suggest that exercise improves both their long-term prospects and their quality of life.

For all of us, the benefits of regular exercise will be improved fitness and reduced fatigue. You may think regular physical activity would increase tiredness and fatigue. Ask anyone who takes regular exercise and they will tell you this is not true. The more we exercise we take, the more energy we seem to have. Indeed, studies show that relaxation actually increases tiredness and fatigue, while a moderate exercise program reduces these symptoms. In addition to increased energy levels, exercise can also play a major role in relieving depression and anxiety. Many studies have shown that regular exercise can:

- increase levels of HDL in our blood
- lower high blood pressure
- help improve body composition by burning fat
- promote lower blood sugar levels
- increase bone density
- boost the immune system
- improve mood and reduce depression.

172

How to assess fitness level and training requirements

Traditionally the BMI or basal metabolic index has been used to indicate one's state of health and level of body fat. It is calculated by dividing your weight in kilograms by your height in metres squared. The acceptable range is 20–25. Obesity is taken to start at a BMI of 30 and gross obesity at 40. A BMI of 18–20 is defined as mild starvation and severe starvation begins when BMI falls below 16. However, it is now acknowledged that the BMI is an inaccurate measure of fitness. For example, a heavily muscled, highly athletic individual will have a high BMI, suggesting unhealthy obesity.

Abdominal obesity is now an acknowledged risk factor for diabetes, heart disease and certain forms of cancer. Dr Margaret Ashwell has developed a simple measure of height versus waist circumference (shown in the Ashwell shape chart, Figure 8). This method can be used to determine the health risk attached to your own shape, i.e. the extent of abdominal obesity, and has been validated by research within the Universities of Cambridge and London. Ideally, your waist measurement should be no more than half your height. Another valuable indicator of overweight risk is the waist to hip ratio, which should be around 0.85 for women and 0.95 for men.

Calculation of your maximum heart rate is necessary before your exercise regime can be designed. This is a simplification but is very useful. It involves the simple sum of subtracting your age in years from the value 220. For example, if you are 60 years old, then $220 - 60 = 160$. This is your maximum heart rate (MHR) and you should not overexert yourself to induce your heart rate to rise above 160 beats per minute. It therefore follows that a 20 year old can exercise to a MHR of 200bpm.

Now we can consider the different exercise regimes in terms of percentages of the MHR. For example, the moderate activity range is 40–60% MHR. Where your activity level falls in this range will depend on your fitness and can easily be calculated by taking your pulse rate at intervals through various exercise regimes. Following illness or prolonged inactivity, you would obviously start at the bottom of this range or lower and gradually work up to 60%. This is where joining a gym and gaining advice from health professionals is crucial. Another bonus is the presence of other like-minded individuals who can offer companionship, moral support and encouragement.

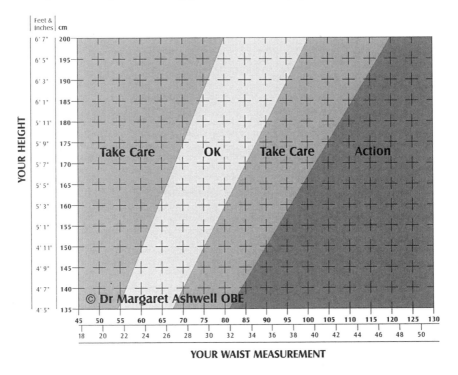

Figure 8 **Ashwell shape chart.**

174

If you are ill or convalescing, there is a performance scale that you can use in agreement with your doctor. It is called the Karnofsky Scale and gives the following fitness ratings that can be used to design exercise programmes (Table 10).

The 70–100% categories can be considered together and can start with 15 minutes of aerobic exercise per day to raise the heart beat to between 60–80% of the MHR. The 10 minute exercise time should be increased by 1–2 minutes per day until a maximum of 40 minutes per session is reached for at least five days per week. A reasonable time to reach the maximum would be about two months. Those in the 50–70% categories must begin with a gentler regime of five minutes three times per day at 55% of their MHR, adding one minute per day to each exercise session

Table 10 **Karnofsky Performance Scale**

Fitness scale	Indicators
100%	No evidence of disease
90%	Normal activity but minor signs of disease
80%	Normal activity with effort and signs of disease
70%	Unable to carry out normal activities but not requiring carers
60%	Requires part-time carers
50%	Frequent medical care and substantial assistance required
40%	Disabled requiring full-time special care.
30%	Severe disability with possible hospitalisation
20%	Extremely ill requiring hospitalisation for treatment
10%	Moribund

until periods are reached, i.e. a total of 30 minutes per day. The sessions are then reduced to two per day and the times extended by a minute per day to a maximum of 15 minutes, again to a total of 30 minutes exercise per day. The final phase involves a reduction to one session per day, i.e. 15 minutes which is then gradually increased to a total of 40 minutes. The final stage will be the ability to maintain an exercise routine at 80% of the MHR for 40 minutes per day. This is a very sensible and safe way to gradually improve fitness. It can take more or less time depending on how rapidly your pulse rate returns to normal after each exercise session. If your pulse rate drops to normal in less than a minute after the workout, then you are ready to progress to the next stage. If not, then persevere at your current level until your recovery improves.

Some form of physical activity every day, consisting of least 30 minutes of moderate intensity aerobic endurance activity, will greatly benefit the health of older individuals [190]. Walk instead of driving short distances. Take the stairs instead of using the elevator or escalator. Other forms of exercise that many of us might not expect to have much health benefit include working on the car or cleaning the house. Participating regularly in some type of physical recreation is even better. Always remember that an active lifestyle is always better than exercise in improving personal health and fitness. Instead of thinking in terms of a specific exercise program, work towards a permanently changed lifestyle to incorporate more activity. Do not forget that muscles used in any activity, any time of day, will contribute to fitness. Conversely, illness and associated bed rest lead to a rapid loss of muscle mass and cardiovascular fitness. It is crucial for convalescing patients to undertake supervised anaerobic resistance training to rebuild the wasted muscle, in addition to aerobic endurance exercise.

If you are seriously ill or incapacitated, you may lack the will to exercise, so a useful alternative to initiate muscle recovery could be the use of devices which use electrical stimuli to cause muscle contraction. There are a variety of inexpensive machines on the market which are sold mainly to health-conscious customers who wish to improve their figures and posture by muscle control. Many years ago during the Korean war, a study was carried out using these devices on US marines who were confined to foxholes with no room for normal exercise. At the end of the study after several days they were found to have increased their muscle strength by up to 40% without any traditional exercise. Normally this kind of inactivity would have led to muscle wasting and loss of strength.

Non exercise activity thermogenesis (NEAT)

If you are overweight, you may have noticed that some of your friends have the irritating ability to eat what they like, do little extra exercise, but never seem to put on weight. You may also have noticed that these friends also have the annoying habit of never seeming to relax and are very fidgety. Could this be a clue to their ability to eat heartily while staying slim? Recent research in the US explains this phenomenon. A 10 year study at the Mayo Clinic involving 150 volunteers has demonstrated some people remain slim because they never really relax physically. In particular they fidget and do not lounge around or sit still for very long. Many obese people on the other hand sit down for an average of 150 minutes longer per day than even the laziest lean people. The slim subjects were found to have a high level of NEAT or non exercise activity thermogenesis, i.e. the ability to burn more calories during everyday activities than obese subjects. The obese subjects had a low level of NEAT and a biological need to sit down for longer. This phenomenon is now thought to be more important than heavy exercise regimes as a means of weight control. You just have to remember never to sit still for more than a few seconds without wriggling, stretching and contracting your major muscle groups.

Remember that an active lifestyle is always better than specific exercise in improving personal health and fitness. Generally, two forms of physical exercise can be performed: these are aerobic and anaerobic exercise, which affect the different types of fibres in our muscles, described below.

Basic muscle structure

Most muscles contain three different types of fibres, which enable them to respond to different requirements from short-term, high intensity activity as in weight lifting and sprinting, to long-term, low intensity activity exercise such as long distance running. All these fibres contract by splitting ATP, the body's most important high energy compound.

Type 1 red fibres

Type 1 red fibres, also referred to as slow oxidative, slow twitch or fatigue resistant fibres, have a rich blood supply and a high myoglobin content to trap the delivered oxygen for aerobic respiration in the mitochondrial-rich fibres. These fibres contract slowly fuelled by the slow utilisation of ATP, which is generated by the mitochondria and involves coenzyme Q10. These fibres are very resistant to fatigue and predominate in the large postural muscles. They play a major role in endurance exercise.

Type 2A red fibres

These are fast oxidative or fast twitch A fibres with some fatigue resistance. They have a very similar rich blood supply, myoglobin and mitochondrial content to Type 1 fibres, but they differ in their high capacity for aerobic ATP generation, again involving coenzyme Q10. Fast ATP utilisation is coupled with rapid muscle contraction. Resistance to fatigue is less than in Type 1 fibres. These fibres play an important role in activities such as swimming and middle distance running.

Type 2B white fibres

Type 2B fibres are also referred to as fast twitch B or fatigable fibres. They have a limited blood supply, a low myoglobin content and few mitochondria. A high glycogen content provides the fuel for anaerobic (glycolytic) ATP synthesis. ATP is rapidly utilised and lactate accumulates to cause early fatigue. These fibres are crucial in short-term power events such as weight lifting and sprinting.

Aerobic exercise

Aerobic exercise is the physical exercise on which most people need to concentrate; it tends to have a long duration, but is usually of low intensity. It should leave us feeling that we have put effort into our exercising with the heart beating faster and breathing stimulated. As a result, there will be an improvement in the efficiency of the heart (slower resting heart rate as the heart muscle becomes stronger) and lungs (slower breathing as the lungs become more powerful). This form of exercise will help to control weight and play a role in increasing muscle and joint flexibility. Participating in any form of aerobic exercise is generally a good idea and will improve health and fitness.

Many different forms of activity involve aerobic exercise. We will all have different requirements and abilities and often practical reasons may prevent us from performing certain exercises. However, most people can do some form of aerobic exercise, even if it is just an exercise as fundamental as walking.

Some common examples of aerobic activities include: aerobics classes, bicycling, brisk walking, football, skiing, dancing, hiking, jogging, skipping, roller skating, running, tennis, squash, stair climbing, stationary cycling, swimming and rowing; these last three exercises are particularly relevant for people with joint problems.

Anaerobic exercise

Anaerobic activities are usually much shorter in duration and emphasise the building of muscle, rather than improving heart rate and breathing rate. Some common examples of anaerobic activities include: football, sit-ups, sprinting and weight lifting.

Which form of exercise provides the greatest health benefits? Aerobic and anaerobic exercise will benefit us greatly, both now and in later years. Ideally we should strive to partake in both forms of exercise as often as possible. The benefits of aerobic exercise appear fairly obvious, while the benefits of anaerobic exercise may not be as apparent. Anaerobic exercise can provide us with a number of vitally important health benefits.

Maintain or enhance lean muscle

With age, muscle mass is lost [230]; in fact we can lose up to half a pound of muscle for each year over 20. This does not sound much, but at age 40, 10 pounds of muscle may have been lost and replaced by body fat, even when consuming a healthy diet. This muscle loss can be reduced/prevented by incorporating some form of anaerobic exercise into the daily routine.

Prevention of injury and increased capacity

The strengthening of the major muscle groups will play a role in diminishing the stress of impact of many daily activities. Strong muscles will help us to do most daily tasks with ease and efficiency. Daily activities such as climbing stairs, getting out of bed, lifting groceries, cleaning the house and mowing the lawn all become easier to do. It is becoming increasingly apparent that footwear and in particular highly cushioned trainers may be having the opposite effect to that which the manufacturers specify in terms of comfort and protection. Biomechanics experts now suggest that the 52 bones in the foot are squashed by trainers. Cushioning makes the foot more unstable, causing the foot to hit the ground on the outside edge of the heel and then roll inwards. This is referred to as 'pronation' and is thought to be responsible for the development of Achilles tendonitis, anterior knee pain and iliotibial band injury (runner's knee). Man evolved to run barefoot, landing softly on the forefoot with the knees flexing to absorb the shock.

Many athletes have found these symptoms to disappear when they start barefoot training, and often suggest that barefoot running on sandy beaches and sand dunes is the best way to start. Caution is of the essence after a lifetime of wearing constrictive footwear which will have weakened the tendons and muscles of the feet. The training build-up needs to be very gradual. If no beaches are available, then grassy soft ground is better than pavements. Anecdotal evidence suggests that this type of training can at least reduce the pain associated with arthritis of the ankles, knees and hips. It is now possible to buy lightweight running shoes with very thin flexible soles to allow the benefits of bare foot running without damage to the feet.

If the weather and outside conditions do not permit barefoot training, then one can train inside on stairs. By standing with the balls of the feet on the edge of a stair, the heels can be slowly lowered and raised to exercise the muscles and tendons in the foot. When the feet are more supple and stronger, the exercises can be repeated one leg at a time and finally wearing a heavy rucksack to increase foot and leg strength even further.

Prevention of osteoporosis

Most anaerobic activities are load bearing exercises. This form of exercise will promote bone growth and calcium deposition in bones. We may not appreciate the importance of this whilst young. However, bone density and calcium deposition in bones will become a major issue with age. This is a particular problem with postmenopausal women. Just as regular workouts build muscle, they also maintain and may even increase bone strength. Strengthening muscles and bones and improving balance can reduce the risk of falls and resulting fractures [231]. Anaerobic exercise will improve health and fitness and is vital for maintaining independence in old age.

So, regular exercise is a good idea for general health and quality of life for both young and old. Regular physical exercise can play a role in prevention of chronic disease such as diabetes, obesity, heart disease and cancer.

Exercise recommendations

The importance of exercise in the prevention and cure of the above conditions cannot be over-emphasised. A combination of high calorie junk food diets and lack of exercise is putting a large section of the population at high risk from these complaints.

On average the extra 5,600 calories from sugar that we may consume per week will require additional exercise of some eight hours (e.g. brisk walking) per week if we are not to put on one extra pound of fat, i.e. 5,600 calories can either support eight hours of vigorous exercise or give rise to 1lb of fat. Clearly, it would be wise to forgo the extra sugary calories unless one can be sure to set aside the vital time for regular brisk exercise.

Many people are dissuaded from vigorous exercise because of injury, disease and/or obesity. Injury or excessive wear, particularly to the knees, hips or ankles (as in osteoarthritis), can severely limit mobility, and immobility further exacerbates these conditions.

One of the best sports for improving whole body fitness and cardiovascular tone is cross country skiing. This incredibly energetic sport is probably beyond most 'armchair athletes', and there is no chance if you live in the UK with the mild winters. However, we can learn from what these skiers do to maintain fitness in milder weather. They exchange their skis/boots for trainers, keep their poles and indulge in vigorous pole-assisted walking. This serves several very important purposes. It spreads the weight load and takes the pressure off sensitive hips, knees or ankles. It improves posture and exercises the upper body muscles. Up to 20% more energy is consumed during fitness resistance walking (FRW) than walking normally at the same speed. Interestingly, although walking at the same speed as normal and expending more energy, FRW actually feels easier. For people who are not desperately keen on too much exercise, FRW could be the perfect solution and we predict that it will become increasingly popular in the future. The advantage of FRW is particularly obvious when attempting to briskly climb steep hills. Normally fatigue rapidly sets in with lack of breath and aching legs. With FRW, because the work load is spread between the legs and shoulders, the blood supply is able to supply the energy needs of the muscles for longer, thus delaying the onset of fatigue. Moreover, the descent is much less stressful on the knees, when the poles are used to take the weight off the knees and increase the points of contact.

Cycling is a long established form of exercise which particularly suits those with damaged joints who can no longer run and the regime can be very accurately tailored to suit various levels of fitness and mobility. Jane Tomlinson, the amateur English athlete, carried out a series of athletic challenges while suffering from disseminated cancer, and raised £1.85 million for charity. In 2000 her doctors gave her 12 months to live, but this courageous woman survived for a further six years. In 2006 she cycled 3800 miles across the US and raised £250,000.

Swimming is an excellent way of improving cardiovascular health without damaging the joints. Bad weather is a big disincentive to outdoor exercise, but this can be overcome by joining a gym, where you can obtain professional advice on training regimes to suit your particular needs on a year round basis which is crucial.

If you are a cancer patient, then the sauna has added value as many tumours are heat sensitive and can regress with repeated sauna sessions. However, the same is not true for heart patients who may be at increased risk in sauna temperatures.

The absolute minimum time for useful exercise

Recent research indicates that it is possible to maintain a basal level of fitness and cardiovascular health with a basic minimum of four minutes vigorous exercise per day at 80% of your MHR. Your pulse rate is best measured by wearing a wrist pulse recorder. You can then get a precise measure of pulse rate and calories burned. When you have found out how many calories per minute you need to expend, you can then use rowing machines, treadmills and steppers in the gym which usually give you an accurate readout of your calorie expenditure. Apparently the best approach is to break your four minute session into six, 40-second periods of exercise with intervening 20 second rest periods.

It must be emphasised that this regime is only to maintain a basal level of fitness and will not be sufficient to result in significant weight loss. As we have already stressed, obesity, diabetes, CHD and cancer are by far the greatest causes of death in the developed world, where unhealthy calorie-rich diets are consumed and levels of exercise are inadequate. The good news is that the same lifestyle changes can protect against, or reverse, all of these conditions.

Excessive exercise can damage your health

Having extolled the virtues of sensible exercise, the opposite scenario must be discussed. Sometimes unfit people become fixated with exercise as a means of improving their health, and embark on unrealistic training programmes without adequate supervision. This is particularly true where endurance running is chosen as part of a weight loss programme. One common problem is the lack of adequate warm up and cool down routines, resulting in muscle and tendon damage. Another problem is expecting unrealistic levels of improvement and overexerting muscles in the process. Any programme should aim for a gradual steady improvement and will require substantial patience.

When patients experience very positive results from exercise programmes, they are sometimes tempted to move to higher levels of exertion. This needs to be carefully monitored because excessive high intensity exercise, particularly endurance running, can depress the immune system. This is the reason why many top class athletes suffer more infections than the average population. Always take medical advice from your doctor before embarking on any exercise programme and further advice from a qualified fitness instructor will enable you to select the optimum programme for your particular needs.

Exercise and heart disease

Physical inactivity is recognised as a major risk factor for coronary artery disease. In fact, the American Heart Association has now added 'lack of exercise' to the list of major risk factors for heart disease. The other risk factors are smoking and high blood pressure. Regular aerobic physical activity increases exercise capacity and plays a role in both primary and secondary prevention of CVD [232, 233]. Primary prevention refers to the initial infarction (heart attack), whereas secondary prevention refers to subsequent heart attacks.

Heart attack survivors may think it is too late to start exercising after the event. This is not the case as regular physical activity can substantially help to reduce the risk of having another heart attack. Moderate regular physical activity after a heart attack will greatly improve chances of survival. Moderate physical activity following a sedentary lifestyle also dramatically reduces the risk of heart attack when undertaken in conjunction with a healthy diet [234, 235].

Exercise recommendations for heart patients

For precise details, the Yale Congestive Heart Failure Programme offers excellent advice. For patients who do not require monitoring during exercise, a walking programme is the best and safest option. One should walk at a comfortable pace some three to four times per week at a speed and for a time that does not result in overexertion. The speed and time should be increased as your fitness improves. If you are initially unsteady or have joint problems, a pair of aluminium telescopic poles can help to increase stability and spread the weight load. You will use more energy but it will feel easier.

Exercise reduces high blood pressure

An analysis of 29 studies aimed at determining the effectiveness of exercise training of four weeks or longer in lowering blood pressure suggested that moderate aerobic exercise had a small but clinically significant effect in reducing systolic and diastolic blood pressure. However, the studies indicated that increasing exercise intensity or increasing exercise frequency to more than three sessions per week did not have any additional impact on reducing blood pressure, but this was in the absence of any dietary control which could yield additional improvements [236].

Exercise increases HDL cholesterol

Endurance trained athletes have much higher HDL cholesterol values compared to sedentary populations [237]. Although it is not yet certain, moderate and high intensity aerobic exercise training appears to be associated with elevated HDL values for both males and females [238, 239]. However, the independent effect of physical exercise and exercise type (aerobic versus resistance training) on total cholesterol, HDL, LDL and TG levels is not fully understood. Results seen may reflect a combination of dietary change and exercise induced loss of body fat. Until more conclusive results are available, we would not recommend using exercise as a sole means of controlling blood cholesterol levels.

Exercise lowers excessive blood glucose levels

Most commonly seen in older people, Type 2 diabetes is associated with insulin resistance and has a combination of risk factors including chronically elevated insulin levels, low HDL, abdominal obesity and high blood pressure. Type 2 diabetes occurs when the body no longer responds to insulin to regulate blood sugar levels as it would do normally. As a result, levels of insulin in the blood become elevated and over time can raise the risk of heart disease [240], as well as kidney failure and blindness. Different exercise regimes can be very effective in the treatment of diabetes. Endurance exercise improves the long-term maintenance of blood glucose levels, while high intensity exercise designed to build up muscle mass increases the activity of muscle glycogen synthase. This allows the body to cope with sudden rises in blood sugar by rapidly converting it to glycogen in the muscles.

Exercise can greatly improve your health in old age

Exercise will develop the blood microcirculation in muscles and this will compete with the blood supply to any tumours present and deprive them of nutrients.

Regular exercise can improve insulin sensitivity in those with insulin resistance and those without. Regular exercise, even a daily walk, requires energy, which is provided by insulin mediated uptake of glucose by cells. As blood sugar levels drop, our body produces less insulin, and this leads to an increased responsiveness by our body to both sugar and insulin. The end result is that insulin sensitivity (a good thing) goes up, which is the opposite of insulin resistance.

Exercise protects against stroke

The evidence of a role for exercise in prevention of CHD in women and men is convincing. The evidence presented for the prevention of stroke with physical exercise has produced more conflicting results. Exercise has been shown to reduce the risk of stroke in some studies [241, 242], but not in others [243, 244]. Vigorous exercise following previous inactivity may dislodge pre-existing arterial plaques, which may block capillaries in the brain, so it would be wise to embark on a healthy diet programme well before the start of any exercise programme in order to allow shrinkage of any plaques. However, the most recent large study suggested that brisk walking and vigorous exercise can have a significant benefit in protection from stroke [245]. This is true for all age groups and in both men and women.

Physical activity is associated with reduced mortality from stroke even after genetic predisposition factors are taken into account. Any physical activity, light, moderate, or heavy, will significantly protect us from stroke. A sedentary lifestyle will increase the likelihood of obesity, high blood pressure and high LDL cholesterol levels, all of which are important risk factors for stroke. One should follow a similar graduated regime as that suggested for heart patients.

Exercise and cancer prevention

Physical activity can have a marked effect upon several functions of the body, and as a consequence affect the chances of cancer development. However, we should stress that the benefits of exercise vary according to the type, frequency, and intensity of the physical activity. Usually, exercise has a positive impact on the cardiovascular system and increases lung capacity and bowel motility. Exercise also helps maintain a healthy immune system, helping regulate hormone levels, antioxidant defence, and DNA repair, all of which reduce the risk of developing cancer.

Regular exercise can help to reduce the incidence of many cancers. Evidence has suggested that high levels of physical activity can help to prevent colon cancer. Exercise has also been seen to help in the prevention of cancers of the breast, prostate, lung and uterus.

The way in which high physical activity may prevent cancer is not clear. There are a number of possibilities, all of which may play a role in reducing cancer risk. Exercise can help reduce obesity, which is related to the cause of several cancers. It can also change the body's hormone levels, which might also have a favourable effect. When exercising, there is an increase in the number of insulin receptors on the surface of cells (non-tumorous), as well as an increase in the sensitivity of the insulin receptors. This will lead to an increased clearance of glucose from the blood as insulin facilitates the transport of glucose into the cells [246]. This process will have the effect of limiting the amount of sugar available for use by tumour cells in the body and may slow down the growth of a tumour and allow time for the immune system to recognise and attack the tumour. Furthermore,

190

exercise stimulates vascular development to the muscle tissues, thus diverting the supply from the cancerous tissue.

Exercise-induced enzyme activity may also play a role in reducing cancer risk. A young healthy adult produces adequate amounts of an enzyme called glycogen synthase. This enzyme converts blood sugar to glycogen and so reduces blood glucose concentrations. Abnormally high blood glucose concentrations can be seen in diabetics and in many cases in the elderly. This is as a result of inadequate activity of this enzyme [247, 248], which is affected by physical activity in that the levels of glycogen synthase will be increased by regular exercise [249]. This suggests that a sedentary lifestyle in addition to ageing may contribute to an increase in blood glucose levels, because of low glycogen synthase levels. Cancer cells have an absolute requirement for glucose in order to grow. Reducing blood glucose levels through exercise may play a crucial role in preventing cancer cell growth. Moreover, vigorously contracting muscles excrete lactic acid as a waste product, as do cancer cells. However, it has recently been demonstrated that relaxing muscle cells can oxidise lactate as an energy source. Cancer cells cannot utilise lactate in this way and are thus further deprived of energy if a patient is very active.

Most research investigating a relationship between exercise and cancer has involved studies of the colon, breast, lung, prostate, testes and endometrium. Of these cancers, the most extensively studied is colon cancer [250, 251].

Exercise and the prevention of colon cancer

Exercise speeds up metabolism and is generally believed to speed up the movement of foods through the colon. This will reduce the time that the colonic mucosal cells (cells that line the colon) are in contact with potential cancer-causing agents which have been consumed. In addition, exercise has a beneficial effect upon the regulation of insulin, prostaglandins and bile acids in the body, all of which have been proved to affect the colon's susceptibility towards cancer development.

Exercise and the prevention of breast and endometrial cancer

Oestrogenic hormones play a role in the development of breast and endometrial cancer. Physical activity may reduce the production, metabolism (breakdown) and excretion of these hormones. Exercise may also reduce the risk of breast cancer through the control of body weight. Indeed, energetic, occupational, leisure and household activities are associated with a reduction in breast cancer rates of 30%, with the highest level of activity producing the greatest reduction in risk [252]. Women who exercise vigorously for about four hours per week can reduce their chances of breast cancer diagnosis by up to 50%.

Exercise and the prevention of prostate cancer

Trained athletes usually show lower levels of circulating testosterone when compared to non-athletes (providing of course, anabolic steroids are not being used). High levels of testosterone have been shown to increase the risk developing prostate cancer. This may represent a potential mechanism, whereby physical activity may protect against prostate cancer by lowering testosterone levels. We use the word 'may' since most, but not all, studies suggest a protective effect [251].

Exercise and cancer treatment

In addition to the function of exercise in the prevention of some cancers, there is a growing interest in the use of physical activity in the treatment and rehabilitation of patients with cancer [253, 254]. A number of studies have suggested that light and moderate exercise, three to five days per week, 20 to 30 minutes per session will have many beneficial effects for people with cancer [255–257]. During cancer treatment, such as surgery, chemotherapy, radiotherapy and hormone therapy, patients may experience a reduced quality of life. Common problems include depression, anxiety and stress [258]. The physical effects of cancer may include ataxia, cachexia (weight loss), reduced cardiovascular and lung function, muscle weakness, fatigue, nausea and pain [259–261]. Fatigue is common and occurs in 40% to 100% of patients undergoing treatment. This may be due in part to the tumour generating lactate. Recent studies have demonstrated that active aerobic muscle can consume lactate, and this will prevent the lactate from being converted to glucose in the liver, thus depriving the tumour of energy.

Regular moderate physical exercise will lead to an increased cardiovascular, lung and muscular function. Other positive effects include improved oxygen consumption, cardiac output, blood supply to muscles, an improved lymphatic circulation, a faster metabolic rate, muscle tone and strength [262]. A review of 24 studies on physical exercise and quality of life following cancer diagnosis published between 1980 and 1997 (most of the studies examined early stage breast cancer and aerobic exercise) concluded that physical exercise has consistent, positive effects upon quality of life for patients, including physical, functional, psychological, and emotional well-being [253]. In fact, over 82% of these studies reported statistically significant positive results. Many of these studies did not involve concurrent dietary optimisation which might have yielded even more impressive results.

General exercise recommendations for cancer patients

Do not attempt any exercise programmes without the agreement of your cancer specialists.

Stage 1. Following surgery/radiotherapy or chemotherapy the patient may be too weak to follow any specified exercise regime. Careful use of faradic muscle stimulation may serve to restore the contractile function so that the patient can then attempt simple limb movements prior to any more demanding regimes.

Stage 2. When patients have recovered sufficiently to get out of bed and walk around the home or the hospital, weights and resistance bands and springs can be used to build up muscle mass and endurance.

Stage 3. Once fully mobile, patients can undertake exercise regimes such as those recommended for recovering heart patients.

Exercise, diabetes and obesity

There are two types of diabetes: Type 1 and Type 2. Type 1 is frequently diagnosed in childhood, and is sometimes referred to as juvenile diabetes for that reason. Type 1 diabetes occurs when the body does not produce any insulin, which is necessary for the body to use sugar. Type 2 is more common and happens when the pancreas does not produce enough insulin or when the body cannot efficiently use the insulin that is produced. The biggest risk factor for developing Type 2 diabetes is being obese (that is, being approximately 20% over your ideal body weight) and over

80% of Type 2 diabetics are obese. Over time, diabetes may cause nerve, kidney and heart damage.

Exercise is an important factor in controlling diabetes. In addition to improving muscle tone and keeping the heart, blood vessels and lungs healthy, increased physical activity will lower blood LDL cholesterol and TG levels (good for hearts) and use calories [263, 264]. This will help those with Type 2 diabetes achieve and maintain an ideal body weight.

Physical activity will also help in controlling diabetes by stimulating insulin secretion, and may reduce the need for medication. Scientific evidence which suggests that regular physical activity can play a role in preventing and reducing the impact of Type 2 diabetes was recently provided by the Diabetes Prevention Program. This was a major research study aimed at discovering whether exercise could prevent or delay the onset of Type 2 diabetes in people with impaired glucose tolerance (those at high risk of developing Type 2 diabetes). Results suggested that regular exercise sharply reduced the chances that such people would develop diabetes [265].

Diabetics usually suffer from abnormally high blood glucose levels, which is indicative of inadequate glycogen synthase activity [266], an enzyme that converts blood glucose into glycogen and so reduces blood glucose levels. This enzyme is regulated by physical activity and is strongly enhanced by both endurance and power exercises [245]. This presents another mechanism by which diabetics can control blood sugar levels.

Just as important are the results of an analysis of controlled clinical trials, which further stress the importance of exercise for people with diabetes. The results of an evaluation of 12 aerobic training studies and two resistance training studies,

195

suggested that exercise reduces sustained high blood sugar levels by an amount that should significantly decrease diabetic complications, such as damage to the kidneys, eyes, heart, nerves and blood vessels [267].

The largest single risk factor for developing Type 2 diabetes is being obese. To most of us, the term 'obesity' means overweight. However, overweight can be defined as an excess amount of body weight that includes muscle, bone, fat, and water. By contrast, obesity specifically refers to an excess of body fat, especially around the stomach.

Abdominal fat is a health hazard

Body fat, particularly in the abdominal region, can no longer be considered as purely a storage depot for fat. Abdominal fat must be considered as an endocrine organ or gland, which produces hormones and inflammatory factors. Moreover, unlike endocrine glands such as the pancreas and adrenals where the size remains relatively constant, abdominal fat can increase in mass often up to 20kg, with a massively increased potential for secreting leptin and the other inflammatory cytokines. The unique metabolism of this tissue underpins the tendency to diabetes, heart disease, arthritis, cancer and other inflammatory diseases in the obese.

Obesity, especially in the abdomen, referred to as central obesity or apple shape, is associated with insulin resistance (a precursor to diabetes), high insulin, elevated blood sugar levels, high cholesterol and blood pressure [268]. These abnormalities lead to Syndrome X, which can lead to diabetes. Regular exercise has been shown to play a role in reversing these abnormalities in people without diabetes [269], suggesting that physical activity could act as a preventative measure against developing diabetes as well as a treatment for obesity.

196

A recent study in the US suggests that the diseases of diabetes and obesity have reached epidemic proportions [270]. Adult obesity rose to 35% in 2012 and is predicted to rise to 42% by 2030. The incidence of diabetes in the US increased by over 49% in only ten years (from 4.9% in 1990 to 7.3% in 2000), with 2,200 new cases diagnosed each day. The Centres for Disease Control and Prevention have predicted that the number of Americans with diabetes will reach 40 million by 2025 [271]. The US is not alone in this problem. In the UK, nearly two thirds of men and over half of all women are now overweight and one in four adults is obese. The level of obesity has tripled in the past 20 years, and is still rising. At the current rate of increase, by 2030 50% of adults will be obese. Obesity is also rising among children. The full magnitude of this problem is revealed in NHS statistics which show a tenfold increase in hospital admissions with a primary diagnosis of obesity for all ages, rising from 1,045 patients in 2000/2001 to 10,571 in 2010/2011.

These statistics are alarming since being overweight, and especially obese, increases the risk of many health problems in addition to diabetes. These include heart disease, certain cancers, stroke, back and joint pain, osteoarthritis, infertility, depression, breathlessness, snoring and sleeping difficulties.

The media generally trivialises the problem of being overweight, suggesting that the only problem is how one will look on the beach or in new clothes. Being obese is not just a cosmetic issue, as many television, magazine articles and adverts would have us believe: it is a serious health issue. Obesity-related disease is a major cause of premature death. In fact, a report from the US National Audit Office concluded that obesity can reduce the average lifespan by nine years.

Exercise has been shown to reduce the risk of development of many chronic diseases. However, this is usually not the reason we exercise. We exercise because it makes us feel better, and for most of us it helps keep our weight under control. It is also one of the best treatments for insomnia and reducing insulin resistance, and a proven aid in the treatment of depression.

It has long been known that obesity predisposes subjects to increased risk of cancer. Obese subjects secrete higher levels of leptin compared to normal people but have become resistant to its suppression of appetite. Recent research has shown that leptin stimulates tumour cells to grow more rapidly.

The multiple roles of leptin

Leptin is synthesised in white adipose tissue, and was initially described as an anti-obesity hormone, since it regulates the balance between food uptake and energy expenditure, by signalling to the brain via the hypothalamus. Thus the changes in stored energy are sensed, and serum leptin concentrations correlate directly with body fat stores. In tandem with insulin, leptin levels fall during starvation and insulin has been shown to stimulate leptin secretion during feeding. Leptin in turn acts upon the pancreas to reduce the secretion of insulin.

Early studies using genetically modified obese mice showed that leptin administration caused a reduction in appetite and weight loss. Unfortunately this effect was not reproduced in studies with obese humans. Overweight and obese people appear to have a resistance to leptin rather like insulin resistance in Syndrome X patients and diabetics, and all the above conditions show varying increases in the level of the proinflammatory C reactive protein (CRP), which is strongly associated with the development of heart disease.

Blood leptin estimation is relatively simple and provides a much better measure of body fat than the body mass index (BMI) as people with the same BMI can have widely different amounts of body fat, e.g. a heavyweight Olympic wrestler versus a couch potato of the same height and weight.

Leptin plays a crucial role in the metabolism of healthy individuals. It controls not only appetite and body weight, but the formation of blood cells, heat generation (maintenance of the body temperature or thermogenesis), reproduction, the growth of new blood vessels (angiogenesis), and the optimisation of the immune system. On the other hand, chronic obesity results from resistance to leptin, which in turn is caused by chronic low-grade inflammation that is associated with obesity. This leads to a vicious cycle of weight gain–inflammation leptin resistance increasing obesity, and can only be broken by substantial weight loss on a prescribed anti-inflammatory diet.

Exercise for diabetics

Exercise programmes must be undertaken with the close supervision of a doctor, to optimise an integrated regime of diet, exercise and medication, to reduce heart disease risk and improve blood glucose regulation. There are special problems associated with exercise routines for both Type 1 insulin dependent diabetes mellitus (IDDM) and Type 2 non insulin dependent diabetes mellitus (NIDDM) diabetics:

- The timing of the exercise

- The amount of insulin injected

- The site of injection.

A regular pattern of diet, exercise and insulin dosage has to be established, with the patient performing an exercise routine within one hour of consuming a meal or snack. The main problem for NIDDM diabetics is weight loss and control. Weight loss through diet and exercise can enable these patients to reduce the amount of oral insulin medication required. Long duration endurance exercise at lower intensity is the best option for NIDDM diabetics.

For both diabetic types, insulin should not be injected into the exercising muscle as this will hasten the onset of hypoglycaemia. Blood glucose levels should be frequently checked and diabetics should always carry supplies of fast acting carbohydrates like juice or sweets, to prevent the onset of hypoglycaemia. Exercise should be avoided during peaks of insulin activity and sugary snacks should be consumed shortly before and during prolonged exercise.

As a result of high blood sugar and poor peripheral circulation, diabetics are particularly prone to the development of diabetic ulcers as a result of minor foot injuries, and should take great care in selecting the best training shoes.

Simple exercise regimes as for the heart and cancer patients can be used, starting at 50–60% MHR and working up to 60–70% for four to seven days per week. Patients with IDDM only require exercise for 20–30 minutes per session. For NIDDM patients, a minimum of 40–60 minutes/day is recommended, starting the programme with 150 minutes/week of moderate intensity activity (50–70% MHR), or with more vigorous activity 90 minutes/week at greater than 70% MHR. The routine should stretch over three days with no more than two consecutive days without exercise.

Vigorous exercise is a very effective way of regulating blood glucose levels. Recent research has defined a simple exercise regime to stabilise blood glucose levels in diabetic patients who are capable of vigorous physical activity. Exercise should not proceed if the blood glucose values are either below 70mg/dl or above 150mg/dl.

For long-term maintenance of major weight loss (13.6kg/30lb), seven hours per week of moderately to vigorous aerobic exercise would be required. NIDDM patients should also be encouraged to weight lift in order to increase muscle mass which will improve their glucose clearance. This, however, will not result in any weight loss.

Recommendations for the overweight, obese and non-diabetic

These categories can be considered together, with the exception of morbidly obese patients, as they are more robust and capable of making great improvements on strict exercise/diet regimes. However, since medical studies on obesity rarely achieve better than 50% compliance, it is easy to see why pharmaceutical alternatives appear so attractive to the medical profession, and to the patients.

While studies have shown that 150 minutes/week of moderate intensity exercise can greatly improve health, much longer sessions are required for long-term weight loss. Two studies with overweight and obese women indicated that a total of 350–450 minutes/week was required. These studies and many others indicate that optimum weight loss and health maintenance require about an hour of moderate intensity activity per day with sensible dietary modification.

In conclusion, the obesity epidemic that is already well advanced in Britain and the US threatens to overwhelm the already overstretched health services with dire consequences. Recent research is predicting the horrific scenario of current parents outliving their children. It is incumbent upon every one of us to pressure our political representatives, to have the courage to restrain the antisocial activities of the all-powerful food and pharmaceutical industries. Nothing will be achieved until young children can be weaned off the addictive junk foods and drink that form a major part of current diets, and adequate sport and exercise becomes a mandatory part of the school curriculum.

Stress and stress management

The main purpose of this book is to discuss the role of diet and exercise in health maintenance. However, it is becoming increasingly apparent that stress plays a major role in the development of cancer, heart disease, obesity and diabetes as well as many other ailments, including several mental illnesses. Since we are not qualified psychotherapists, we will try to restrict our comments to the biochemical basis of stress and its management.

The most striking examples of how stress in populations can increase heart disease can be found in the book *The Great Cholesterol Con* by Dr Malcolm Kendrick. He effectively debunks the cholesterol theory of heart disease with numerous examples of epidemiological studies from impeccable sources.

Metabolism can be divided into the processes of anabolism (synthesis and storage) and catabolism (breakdown of energy reserves and release of energy). Anabolism is associated with digestion of food, uptake of nutrients and synthesis of body tissues, under conditions of minimal stress. Catabolism, on the other hand, is stimulated by stress and initiates a series of reactions that provide the body with energy sources to overcome the physical aspects of stress (fight or flight responses).

Both these pathways are controlled by different parts of the autonomic nervous system which is not under our conscious control. These are the parasympathetic and the sympathetic nervous systems. The adrenal gland is considered as part of the sympathetic nervous system. Both systems are referred to as the hypothalamic–pituitary–adrenal axis or HPA axis for short. Table 11 demonstrates how higher animals (including humans) have evolved a beautiful, intricate nervous system to enable a healthy

Table 11   **Some functions of the autonomic nervous system**

Parasympathetic	Sympathetic
Decreases heartbeat	Increases heartbeat
Constricts bronchi	Dilates bronchi
Stimulates bile secretion from liver	Stops glycogen synthesis in liver
Initiates cephalic phase of digestion from sight and/or smell of food	Stimulates glucose production
	Triggers release of blood clotting factors
Increases secretion from salivary glands	Decreases digestive secretions
Stomach and pancreas activation	Increases sweat gland secretions
Gut sphincter relaxation	Gut sphincter contraction
Urinary bladder wall contraction	Urinary bladder wall relaxation

response to intermittent periods of stress. If, however, the stress is continuous, then recovery is severely inhibited and the balance of the HPA axis becomes disturbed. This is often referred to as HPA axis dysfunction.

How persistent stress leads to obesity, diabetes and heart disease

The anabolic reactions controlled by the parasympathetic nervous system are crucial for recovery, following reaction to stress. They cannot occur effectively if the sympathetic system is consistently activated, even by low levels of stress. When both pathways are activated simultaneously, the body tissues and organs receive conflicting signals, e.g. the simultaneous presence of insulin, adrenaline and cortisol disrupts the processes involved in the storage and release of glucose and lipids. Blood glucose levels rise, followed by insulin. Fat mobilisation and synthesis is stimulated followed by deposition on artery walls and the redistribution of peripheral fat to the abdominal (visceral) region. Visceral fat deposition, also referred to as central obesity, is a major risk factor for both diabetes and heart disease. Couple this with the increased heart rate, blood pressure and clotting factors in the blood and the risk of heart disease becomes obvious.

In the developed and developing countries, the epidemic increases in obesity and Type 2 diabetes appear to be related to unhealthy diets, lack of exercise and stress, where 'comfort' eating may be a response to stress, particularly among the disenfranchised. This is because cortisol, released during stress, stimulates areas of the brain concerned with the pleasurable sensations related to sugar and fatty food consumption. This long-term effect of cortisol represents a state of chronic stress. In contrast, the short-term healthy effects of cortisol stimulate glucose release for energy metabolism in healthy individuals. Furthermore, recent research links stress with sleep deficit and central obesity.

Psychological rather than physical stress should not be underestimated as a potent risk factor. Feelings of lack of worth or inadequacy can lead to long-term stress and ill health. One may have a feeling of lack of control over one's life, e.g. working hard and doing an excellent job only to find your superior taking all the credit for your ideas and denigrating you in front of his/her superiors. If you cannot move jobs, this type of situation can trigger coronary lipid deposition and visceral fat deposition and immune suppression due to increased levels of cortisol. Recent surveys have shown that top politicians and executives holding high office rarely succumb to this type of stress.

Chronic stress can result in hyper-secretion of cortisol, which desensitises immune cells and will reduce their capacity to respond to cortisol. As a result, inflammatory processes can take place. This non-specific inflammation induced by immune cells may contribute to diseases involving such reactions, such as heart disease, multiple sclerosis and rheumatoid arthritis [272].

One of the worst examples of psychological stress and related diseases must be the case of the Australian Aborigines. Living in an affluent country, they have the lowest living standard of anywhere in the world. Poverty, unemployment and poor educational attainment are typical and coupled with high incidence of abdominal obesity, diabetes and heart disease.

Other factors supporting the role of psychological stress in degenerative diseases are the many large population studies showing a link between social dislocation and heart disease. This was seen following the mass immigration to the US during the early 1900s. The stress-related effects upon public health of socio-economic change following de-urbanisation, de-industrialisation and deregulation of the food industry in the 1970s and 1980s, in conjunction with poor nutrition, underpins the current US obesity epidemic [273]. Other examples of population stress include large-scale repatriation (Finland, 1948), and the collapse of the social fabric and health provision in post-communist Russia, where life expectancy is now 20 years less than it was in 1990. Similar problems have arisen in the ex-satellite countries following the break-up of the USSR. In contrast, there are the low levels of cardiovascular disease in France and Spain, where the Mediterranean ethos appears to yield a healthy separation between stress and relaxation. The question of general health should also be considered with respect to stress, when high cortisol levels depress the immune system. This property of corticosteroids is used to advantage in transplant and graft operations, where administered corticoids are used to suppress the immune response and prevent tissue rejection. Sustained secretion of corticosteroid hormones also results in a stimulation of vascular calcification which adds to the risk of lipid associated CVD.

We can contrast the adult stress scenario with the problems of stress/poverty and childhood obesity. It is now well established that maternal stress and poor nutrition during pregnancy can have detrimental effects upon the foetus, leading to reduced growth in utero and low birth weight. Subsequent rapid growth of the underweight infant with adequate nutrition often leads to development of obesity. The converse is not true for maternal obesity, which often leads to overweight progeny with an increased risk of obesity and Type 2 diabetes in later life. Maternal smoking, often due to stress, will further damage the foetus because of a lack of oxygen supply. The above suggests that the public conception of obesity as a lack of personal will power should be questioned. Rather, obesity in many instances is probably rooted in infancy and childhood, when strong genetic and imposed environmental determinants such as stress can shape a still developing child.

Can you die from a broken heart? This romantic notion does in fact have a scientific basis. Recent research has shown that sudden emotional stress can trigger a severe but reversible heart muscle weakness that mimics a heart attack. During times of such stress, a large amount of adrenalin and similar catecholamines are released into the bloodstream. This sudden and often overwhelming stress releases such a flood of these chemicals that the heart muscle is stunned. Early treatment can reverse this effect with no lasting damage.

Stress and ageing

For many years the major adrenal steroid hormone, dehydro-epiandrosterone (DHEA) and its sulphate had no known function. During the past 20 years, research has shown that this multifunctional steroid has many important biochemical roles. In adolescent children, it has a crucial role as an androgen (male sex hormone) precursor in the peripheral tissues and plays a vital role in growth and development. It reaches a peak at around 25 years and thereafter serum levels decrease at a rate of about 2% per year. At 80 years the serum level is virtually zero. This may be the main reason why older people are less able to cope with stress. Several recent publications indicate that serum levels of DHEA vary considerably in a given population and that a healthy, vigorous lifestyle tends to stimulate the continued synthesis of DHEA. Moreover, patient groups with naturally lower serum DHEA levels were found to be less responsive to exercise regimes as a means of stress management than those groups with naturally high or supplemented DHEA. Clinical trials were invariably more successful with subjects over 50 years of age. Negative results with younger subjects (25–35 years) probably indicate that people of this age range are already producing adequate amounts of DHEA.

It should be noted also, that while DHEA levels drop with age, the pattern of cortisol secretion remains relatively constant. This may be a major factor in the reduced immune response and muscle loss often seen in the aged. These suppositions are supported by somewhat patchy evidence and have resulted in DHEA being described as a miracle anti-ageing drug, particularly in the US where DHEA supplementation does not require a prescription. In the UK, the drug can only be obtained following a medical consultation and prescription. Recent research indicates that DHEA levels correlate with the ability to recover from high intensity exercise, (i.e. reduced muscle damage), and resistance to post-exercise infection often seen in top class athletes because of the hyper-secretion of cortisol. For non-elite athletes, it would appear that DHEA supplementation offers the most promise for those over 50 years of age.

DHEA supplementation should not be undertaken, even in the US, without prior medical consultation. Serum levels can vary greatly between individuals and there is some clinical evidence that supplementation can lead to sex hormone imbalances with masculinisation in women and feminisation in men. However, the positive effects of supplementation may outweigh the side effects, particularly in the stressed over 50s, where a blood DHEA determination would be wise council.

9 Renewal, disease prevention and self-help

This chapter outlines the lifestyle changes needed to minimise the risk of the major killer diseases, and the modifications which offer the best chance of reversing the conditions in those already affected. Obesity, diabetes, CHD and cancer are the major causes of death in the developed world where unhealthy calorie-rich diets are consumed, stress levels are high, and exercise is inadequate. The good news is that the same lifestyle changes can protect against all of these conditions.

Whatever your condition, you can give your body a better chance of recovery by following the recommendations in this chapter, whilst referring back to the more detailed information given earlier. Following appropriate lifestyle changes, many people can recover from these major diseases, so if you are suffering there is no reason why you could not become one of them.

Most of us can think of a number of food products eaten every day that may not be good for our health. However, the threat of developing a disease at some time in the future is not enough motivation for most people to eat healthily. The pleasure and convenience of unhealthy foods are the main reasons for their consumption in vast quantities in the Western diet. This is not to say that a healthy diet need be unpleasurable. With a careful stocking of the larder and snack planning, our taste buds need not lose out to our health. However, it has to be said that it will prove almost impossible to eliminate highly processed foods from a 'normal' diet. The secret is to limit the intake of these foods as much as possible.

Dietary sources of healthy calories

What proportion of the healthy food we eat each day should be fat, protein and carbohydrate?

To begin with, we do not agree with the generally accepted daily proportions of carbohydrate, protein and fat consumption recommended for a healthy diet (A), shown in Table 12. Our recommendations (B) show an increased consumption of fat and protein and a reduced consumption of carbohydrates. The amount of carbohydrates consumed per day is reduced by 25%; dietary fat is increased by 20% to a level consumed pre-1950 when the incidence of heart disease and obesity was very low.

When consuming the WHO recommendation of 2500 calories a day (for an average active 70kg man), the actual weight and calories of foods consumed per day using *our* current recommendations would be as follows:

Carbohydrates = 219g (875 calories)
Protein   = 94g   (375 calories)
Fat   = 140g (1,250 calories)

This new recommendation of 35% of total calories consisting of carbohydrate would still be unhealthy if consumed from sugar and white flour in processed foods. Complex carbohydrate is an essential part of a healthy diet.

The level of calorie consumption will obviously vary between individuals. Calories consumed by an average active 60kg woman will be 2100 per day. In both men and women, calorie consumption should be reduced with an inactive lifestyle, if fat deposition is to be avoided. With growing children, calories should be restricted only if there are signs of unhealthy weight

Table 12 **Authors' recommended food proportions**

Nutrient	(A)	(B)	Healthy food sources
Carbohydrates	60%	35%	Complex carbohydrates
Protein	10%	15%	Good quality unprocessed food source
Fat		30%	50%	Medium chain fats (butter and coconut oil)
			Long chain fats (animal sources, palm and olive oils)
			Essential fats (polyunsaturated oils from fish and unrefined flax)

gain. Particularly for children, calories derived from processed foods should be avoided at all costs. Fizzy drinks and high calorie snack foods retard healthy development, especially of the brain.

Portion control

From the outset, the well-known tip of using smaller dining plates to reduce the visual shock of smaller portion sizes will help with portion control. It is useful to visualise a portion size, e.g. 100g of mashed potato or 100g of steak. To do this simply place a plate upon a set of kitchen scales, adjust the scale back to zero and add the appropriate food item in 100g quantities. This allows you to visualise 100g portions of different food types. Thereafter it should be possible to measure correct quantities of food by eye without using scales.

Armed with the knowledge of how many calories and grams of each food type we can consume per day for a healthy diet, we can now look at some healthy alternatives (Table 13).

Table 13   **Calories/100g for a range of foods**

Food	Carbohydrates	Protein	Fat
Butter	0	13.2	740
Cheese (Cheddar)	Trace	100	315.4
Eggs	Trace	50.3	97.6
Milk (whole)	18	13.2	35.6
Yoghurt (plain Greek)	18.6	22.6	91.7
Meat, poultry, fish			
Lean (average)	0	80	120
Fatty (average)	0	63	267
Poultry (lean)	0	112	58
Poultry (fatty)	0	100	231
Fish, white (average)	0	88	12
Fish, oily (average)	0	86	86
Bread (wholemeal)	156.7	35.5	21.5
Oils			
Coconut oil	0	0	891
Olive oil	0	0	891
Palm oil	0	0	891

In this food recommendations chapter, a conscious decision was made not to include the almost obligatory set of recipes. Instead we have chosen to provide a selection of the healthy alternatives described earlier and indicate the number of calories obtained from 100g of each food type. This will give a clear insight as to the source and amount of the calories consumed each day. The individual decides upon the appropriate recipe and the foods contained within. However, we must stress that this is NOT a calorie counting exercise for weight loss, as seen in many popular publications. Rather, what we present here is a guide for individuals to use as a tool when choosing specific food types and amounts to provide, maintain and in many instances regain good health. Some diets require the careful weighing of the various components each day. We suggest that this is too time-consuming and will soon be too tedious to continue. A better approach is to weigh various foods, put them on a plate and get a feel for the appearance of the portion size. Thereafter foods can be dispensed quickly on a basis of their size on the plate. Italian nutritionists use this technique in diet questionnaires with colour pictures of the different meals and portion sizes. With this technique, after the initial effort, foods can be accurately prepared and served with a minimum of effort.

Table 13 is meant as a general guide only. The food sources quoted here are for unprocessed food, and processed foods containing the above foods will contain added and usually unwanted ingredients such as carbohydrates and trans fats. For detailed information, one should consult the Healthy Diet Calorie Counter [274]. Vegetables have not been included in this table. All fresh vegetables are of great beneficial value to health and should be consumed everyday if possible. The only exception to this is the excessive amounts of potatoes and potato chips (invariably cooked in vegetable oil containing trans fats).

213

Similarly, fruit has not been included in the table. With the exception of dates, figs and raisins, all fruits should be consumed daily if possible.

Assessing calorie requirements

Table 14 shows the optimum average daily calorie requirement for moderately active children. Note the lower energy requirements for girls. This is not because they are less robust or active than boys, but that they have a much more efficient energy metabolism, evolved to increase chances of survival through periods of starvation. Table 15 shows the optimum average daily calorie requirements for moderately active adults.

It must be stressed that the values in the tables are averages and can only be used as approximations in calculating your energy requirements. Common sense is crucial and a visit to your doctor will give you details of your healthy body weight for your height and age. For example, it may not be immediately obvious that a tall, thin person with some abdominal fat may be more at risk of CHD than a chubby, small but well-muscled adult

Table 14 **Optimum average daily calorie requirement for moderately active children**

Age (years)	Boys (kcal)	Girls (kcal)
1–3	1250	1175
4–6	1700	1550
7–10	1975	1750
11–14	2225	1850
15–18	2750	2100

with heavy bones. Women who are breastfeeding, who have not gained significant excess weight during pregnancy, will need to increase their calorie intake by about 500kcal per day. Following weaning the normal diet can be resumed. The importance of natural breastfeeding for child brain development cannot be over-emphasised. Supplementation of the pregnant and nursing mother's diet with oily fish or fish oils can greatly improve the baby's brain development.

The rate of development in children can vary enormously and the maintenance of an optimum diet for healthy growth is essential. The increased calorie requirements during growth spurts must be skilfully diverted away from junk foods. Also the development of what is euphemistically called 'puppy fat' should not be allowed to lead to childhood obesity.

In simple terms, if you are overweight then you must reduce your calorie intake by first reducing consumption of the refined carbohydrates found in typical junk foods. Chances of success will be further improved by starting a vigorous exercise regime. If you are underweight, the problem may be more complex and the psychological aspects should be assessed by a specialist doctor. When these have been resolved, a diet and exercise programme must be undertaken with an energy-rich diet

Table 15 **Optimum average daily calorie requirements for moderately active adults**

Age (years)	Men (kcal)	Women (kcal)
19–59	2700	2050
60–75	2350	1900
75+	2100	1800

of protein, fats and complex carbohydrates (corrected for height, weight, age and sex) until you reach your ideal weight. Exercise is crucial for muscle regeneration; otherwise weight gain will be in fat, making you even less inclined to exercise, and increasing your risk of obesity-related diseases.

Using the above tables after calculating your BMI (see Chapter 8) you should be able to devise a diet to either modify or maintain your body weight. Use the calorie tables to source healthy foods from which to derive your daily calorie intake. We suggest a ratio of 50% fat: 15% protein: 35% carbohydrate. Your daily fat intake should comprise of 70g Saturated fat (preferably the shorter chain fats found in butter and coconut oils), 70g monounsaturated fat and 1g omega 3 fat.

Marine fish and cod liver oil can be taken as capsules if oily fish are not a regular part of the diet. For non-vegetarians, fish and krill oils are the best option because they are rapidly absorbed and converted directly into essential metabolites. Hemp and flax oils require additional reactions and conversion to the useful end-products is much less efficient. Vegetarians are advised to source algal products which contain the same long chain omega-3 fats as fish oils.

Cardiovascular disease: heart attack risk factors

- Stress and depression can triple the risk in both sexes.
- Increased blood pressure (hypertension) can triple the risk for men and double it for women.

- Smoking may double or triple the risk depending on other lifestyle factors such as poor diet and lack of exercise.
- A high LDL/HDL ratio is associated with a quadrupling of risk but only in association with a cluster of lifestyle risk factors such as smoking.
- Abdominal obesity, even in otherwise slim individuals, doubles the risk.
- Eliminating 'junk' foods in favour of healthy whole foods can reduce the risk by some 30%.
- Lack of exercise increases risk by a minimum of 20%.

A quick perusal of the above list should be a potent wake-up call, particularly if more than one of the above high risk factors is applicable to you. Immediate medical advice and remedial action is imperative.

Your heart and how to protect it

The heart is a unique organ and only stops beating when you are dead. It is amazingly resilient and you may have wondered why it is that you have not heard of many people dying of heart cancer. Could it be that the constant activity prevents the cancer taking hold and does this give us a clue as to the value of exercise in preventing and/or curing other cancers?

The heart is, however, extremely susceptible to lack of blood sugar and oxygen, which gives rise to the classic symptoms of a myocardial infarction or heart attack. Patients may suffer a series of minor heart attacks culminating in a fatal event. If early warning signals are heeded and the appropriate action taken, subsequent attacks can be prevented and the quality of life significantly enhanced. If you have had heart bypass surgery, your subsequent diet and exercise regimes will be crucial. Your damaged arteries may have been replaced with veins which have much thinner walls and are much less robust, and require regular and sustained exercise to stimulate their muscle wall development. This enables them to perform more like arteries in supplying an adequate supply of blood to the heart. Also a healthy diet and reduced stress will prevent the re-occurrence of the conditions that led to your operation in the first place.

How a combination of factors exacerbates heart problems

Imagine this scenario. Following a stressful day at the workplace, a man is caught in a traffic jam on his way home. He arrives home late and rushes a convenience food dinner (high in refined carbohydrate, ITFs and salt) in order to watch his football team on TV. With a high carb beer and a cigarette/cigar, he goes on to watch his team get beaten by a normally third rate opposition.

These factors combine to produce a significantly higher risk through the following process:

1. Stress at the workplace and in the traffic jam stimulates the release of the glucocorticoid hormones, which raise the blood sugar and cause muscle breakdown. The stress hormone adrenaline (epinephrine) is also released which stimulates the release of fatty acids into the blood, to provide energy for an energetic response and this results in an elevation of your blood pressure and fat deposition on your artery walls.

2. This situation is exacerbated by inactivity and consumption of junk food. The high carbohydrate and trans fat content of junk food results in more fat

deposition on the artery walls. Along with a high salt intake, this further raises your blood pressure.

3. This is during a period of stressful TV watching. As little energy is expended, more stress hormones are released and blood pressure and blood lipids rise yet again.

4. Toxins from the cigarette/cigar smoke in the blood cause oxidative stress where LDL particles are oxidised and taken up by white blood cells to form foam cells which can then adhere to the artery walls.

Cancer comments on trends and treatment outcomes

Cancer cells are competing with our healthy tissues for nutrients, and in particular glucose because they have a defective metabolism and cannot obtain energy from fat. This gives us two crucial weapons in our natural armoury to either prevent or attack the disease. Sugar and refined carbohydrate can be eliminated from the diet without any ill effects whatsoever.

Exercise has an additional protective effect, because contracting muscles require glucose for energy and diverts it from the tumour cells. Moreover, exercise causes muscles to increase their blood supply, further diverting nutrients from the tumours, and lactate produced by muscle activity may further inhibit tumour growth. This will starve the tumours and may cause them to regress and allow the immune system time to recognise and destroy them before they overwhelm the body. Recent research on low carbohydrate or ketogenic diets indicates that ketones may have at least two very valuable functions. Not only do they inhibit tumour growth but they may also prevent loss of muscle mass in cachexia, which is the cause of death in 40% of terminal cancer patients (see Chapter 3).

This condition mimics the natural response to partial starvation during the night when muscle protein is broken down to maintain blood glucose levels. This process stops naturally during prolonged starvation or when subjects follow a ketogenic Atkins or low GI type diets. This could prove a valuable strategy to combat cancer and cachexia. Ketogenic diets gave spectacular levels of tumour regression and survival whereas the mice on normal carbohydrate rich diets had 100% mortality [41] This ketogenic diet approach to cancer treatment has recently be used in human clinical trials with promising results.

Additional strategies involve consuming vegetables with anti-cancer components such as avocado, chilli peppers and watercress. Chilli peppers contain capsaicin which has been shown to cause some cancer cells to self-destruct. Watercress and other brassicas have dual protective functions. They contain one class of nutraceuticals that activates enzymes in the liver which detoxify carcinogens. The other group interacts directly with tumour cells to cause their destruction. Notice that none of these vegetables contain appreciable amounts of carbohydrates.

General conclusions

Many people and some doctors believe that a low fat, high-carbohydrate diet is healthy. This is encouraged by the numerous slimming organisations that support this opinion. This does not make this opinion correct. Nutritionists at the Harvard School of Public Health have recently publicly criticised this recommendation [228]. These scientists suggested that the food pyramid fails to distinguish between refined and complex carbohydrates and their relative glycaemic responses (level of sugar released into our blood). Further, it was pointed out that there was little evidence to support the dominant nutritional message that diets high in complex carbohydrate promote good health. Neither the food pyramid nor the RDA is based on scientific fact. Following these guidelines you may be at an increased risk of development of degenerative diseases such as diabetes, heart disease, cancer, bowel disease, autoimmune diseases and many more.

Although we give dietary recommendations, what we are really advocating is a lifestyle change. The word diet is most often associated with sacrifice, hunger, guilt and unhappiness. Most diets involve restricting the amount of food consumed in an attempt to reach a given body weight, and this is always accompanied by cravings and feelings of hunger. Common sense should tell us that a calorie controlled diet for weight loss cannot be continued indefinitely. What happens when the diet is over and a goal weight has been reached? We all know the answer. Usually the weight lost is regained and so the cycle begins again. Weight loss will become increasingly difficult with successive cycles, as many people can testify.

In addition to this ultimately unhealthy cycle of weight loss and gain, very little thought is often given to the nutritional aspects of these diets. It is assumed that if we are not overweight, then we must be healthy. This is not true. The type of food we consume will play a greater role in our health than the number of calories consumed. Sacrificing our health for our weight is a bad idea, and calorie restriction should only be attempted if particular attention is paid to the nutritional content of the diet.

221

We must stress that the recommendations made here are not aimed at energy restriction. Rather, we are concerned with advocating a lifestyle that will include a diet which will provide health, protection from chronic diseases and if we are overweight, attainment of a healthy body mass, all at the same time.

Following the dietary recommendations we have put forward will undoubtedly lead to improved health. However improving and maintaining good health does not only involve eating the right food. Regular physical exercise plays just as an important role in our health as the food we eat. Exercise can take many forms and does not necessarily involve enrolment in a gym programme. Regular physical activity enhances our health, aids our recovery from illness and can also play a significant role in protecting us from a range of chronic diseases including diabetes, obesity, heart disease and cancer.

In conclusion, it can be seen that the consumption of a wide variety of fresh fruit and vegetables will provide not only beneficial vitamins, minerals and fibre but associated nutraceuticals that protect against the diseases associated with oxidative stress.

Ten tips for health and combating the big four diseases

1. Stop smoking. Stop smoking to reduce the risk of CHD, lung cancer and bronchitis. Smokers are three to four times more likely to suffer CHD than non-smokers.

2. Take exercise. One hour of brisk exercise per day, or four minutes of intense exercise (80% of maximum heart rate) per day, which is composed of six, 40-second bursts of exercise followed by 20 seconds of intervening rest periods. Those

222

suffering from CHD should seek medical advice before engaging on any exercise regime. More sustained low intensity exercise is required by those on weight reduction regimes.

3.   Eat healthily   Reduce as far as possible the consumption of foods with a high glycaemic load such as sugar, potato, white rice and pasta, and replace these with wholemeal products, or even better, extra green vegetables or cauliflour.   Avoid convenience foods such as sweets, ice creams and pizzas. Avoid comfort eating unhealthy food. Try and eliminate sugar from the diet altogether. This will involve not only eliminating added sugar, but sugar in processed foods and fruit as well. Try using the low GI sugar xylitol as an alternative.

4.   Eat the right fats.   Treat current advice on dietary fat intake with caution. A healthy intake can be 50% of total calories consumed.   For a 70kg male we recommend 70g Saturated fat (preferably the shorter chain fats found in butter and coconut oils), 70g monounsaturated fat and 1g omega 3 fat.
The optimum ratio of omega-6:omega-3 fats should be 1:1. Avoid partially hydrogenated vegetable oils and foods containing them as they add too much omega-6 fat to the diet and stimulate fat storage and inflammation, if the diet is also rich in refined carbohydrates. Avoid the latest 'healthy' butter replacements which contain excess omega-6 fat and insignificant amounts of omega-3 fat from plant sources.

5. *Watch your weight.* Maintain body weight as of 21 years (assuming a healthy physique) with weight increases of no more than 14kg in the absence of serious strenuous exercise.

6. *Eat fruit and vegetables.* Consume fruit and vegetables at least five times per day, with the accent on salads and low sugar fruits. This can reduce the risk of CVD by between 30–50%.

7. *Eat fibre.* Although fruit and vegetables supply some dietary fibre, this should be supplemented with cereal fibre (10g/day) which protects against colon cancer and CVD. Recent research indicates that oats and oat bran supply vitamins and hydrophilic fibre which act to lower LDL cholesterol. Resistant starch in green bananas can help to control blood sugar and stimulate body fat loss.

8. *Watch your alcohol intake.* Alcohol drunk in moderation with no more than one to three units per day, three small whiskies or three half pints of beer, protects against CVD, but needs to be eliminated from weight reduction diets. Alcohol is metabolised preferentially by the tissues, thus diverting calories from fat and carbohydrate to form fat in the adipose tissue.

9. *Include vitamin E.* Even a healthy diet may not contain the level of E vitamins needed to protect against free radical damage from pollutants in the urban environment. Supplement-ation with the chemically produced α-tocopherol is not recommended, even though it is found in the naturally occurring mixture of tocopherols and tocotrienols. A healthier alternative is to use wheat germ, rice bran or unrefined palm oils (one teaspoon per day) which are a rich source of the eight natural vitamin E isomers. The beneficial effects of natural vitamin E supple-

mentation are greatly enhanced when vitamin C (preferably from fruit) and red and purple pigmented fruit and vegetables are consumed simultaneously.

10. Include vitamin C. Healthy subjects on a good diet should obtain adequate vitamin C from their intake of fresh fruit and vegetables. However, people at high risk or suffering from the big four diseases would be well advised to increase their vitamin C intake by supplementation to at least 1g/day. Soluble vitamin C is lost very rapidly in the urine, so the best strategy is to take slow release tablets to prolong the benefits. Vitamin C is absolutely vital for health and works synergistically with the E vitamins and many other dietary antioxidants. It is crucial for the prevention of all the diseases resulting from oxidative stress, and has even been shown to inhibit the growth and spread of tumours, when it has been administered intravenously at very high doses (10g/day).

Recent studies with implications for child health

Dairy products form an important part of children's diets, but their value is now questionable. Over two thirds of the world's increasing maize production is consumed in animal feeds. This increases the ratio of omega-6 to omega-3 fats some fivefold in meat and dairy products when compared to grass-fed cattle or game. This high maize diet leads to increased levels of arachidonic acid in both the fatty tissues and the lean muscle [275]. Dietary studies have shown that even modest consumption of these arachidonate-rich products can stimulate the production of inflammatory prostaglandins and cause increased stickiness in blood platelets [276]. Processed foods such as crispy fish fingers, a children's favourite, undergo a 1,000-fold increase in omega-6 fat content when cooked in vegetable oil, compared to the original fresh fish.

Such diets can raise the overall omega-6:omega-3 ratio to 15:1 and much higher. The preferred ratio is closer to unity [277]. It has also been suggested that childhood deficiency of omega-3 fat increases the risk of developing Type 1 diabetes [278]. The use of low fat diets to reduce childhood obesity should be treated with extreme caution, since these diets have been shown to deplete further the already low levels of omega-3 fats by stimulating their oxidation. Moreover, such diets also reduce the uptake of oil-soluble vitamins and pigments. Many studies, going back to the 1970s, indicate that the actual requirement for essential fatty acids is very low if the diet contains adequate amounts of saturated and monounsaturated fats. In fact, pregnant rodents were able to consume saturated fat as their major energy source in the presence of a small amount of omega-3 fat. The nearest human equivalent would be the traditional Inuit diet. Despite this information, many articles in the popular press invariably name saturated fat as the major hazard in modern diets, with little mention of the role of refined carbohydrates and omega-6 fats as causes of obesity.

The omega-6 fatty acids are inflammatory and adipogenic (fat-storing) via the arachidonic acid cascade, causing damage to blood vessels and lung function [279]. Obese animals and children have higher serum levels of omega-6 fats than healthy controls [280] and the effects of omega-6 fats are more pronounced with a diet rich in refined carbohydrates. Studies with animals indicate that optimum fat quality during pregnancy and lactation can have long-term effects in reducing diseases in adulthood [281]. Increased omega-6:omega-3 ratios in human breast milk worldwide is a potent signal that all these animal studies should be repeated in humans.

The other side of the obesity epidemic coin is the role of sugar and calorific sweeteners. A recent Swedish study has shown that high serum insulin levels in healthy children precedes the progression to becoming overweight [282]. These levels would be further elevated by the consumption of refined carbohydrates, particularly the high fructose syrup in fizzy drinks, leading to increased fat accumulation.

Our final advice would be to replace the junk food in your diet with a wide variety of fresh fruit and vegetables that will provide not only adequate calories but beneficial vitamins, minerals, fibre and associated nutraceuticals that protect against the diseases associated with oxidative stress.

Most of the recommendations in this book are now firmly backed up by extremely sophisticated experiments, which were developed in the decade 1990–2000. These experiments are capable of rapidly detecting hundreds of metabolic changes in cultured cells and whole animals (including humans), following nutritional changes. This new science is known as proteomics. It can also be applied to the investigation of the role of exercise and the human genome in disease susceptibility and its prevention or cure, by detecting which genes have been switched on or off by a particular treatment.

In conclusion, there is now sufficient high quality scientific information to enable individuals and government bodies to make properly educated decisions concerning lifestyle and health choices, and to identify inappropriate foods and drugs. What remains is the extremely difficult task of simplifying all the latest relevant and complex information into a form that can be understood by lay people and politicians. It is then very much up to the informed public to lobby politicians to make sensible proposals to reorganise food and drug production and consumption. Nothing less is acceptable if we are to protect the health and wellbeing of future generations.

Appendix

For this more detailed scientific chapter, the reader requires a basic knowledge of biology and chemistry. The molecular basis of oxidative stress is explained, and we examine the role of free radicals in health and disease. We discuss the ways in which the body's own defence system is supplemented by dietary antioxidants to combat oxidative stress. Non-scientists can skim this chapter for key words which will help them to understand earlier chapters.

The scientific basis of oxidative stress

One of the penalties of having evolved to become a complex air breathing organism is that we are subject to oxygen toxicity. Around 4–6% of the oxygen that we breathe ends up as the potentially toxic free radical (FR) superoxide (see below). In order to survive, all air-breathing creatures have evolved mechanisms to detoxify superoxide. Oxidative stress occurs when the ability of the organism to detoxify this and other FRs is overloaded and cellular damage occurs (Figure 9).

Free radicals

Free radicals are molecules or atoms that possess one or more unpaired electrons, are extremely reactive, and short-lived. They damage biological molecules in their close proximity. Most of the biologically relevant free radicals contain oxygen atoms.

Reactive oxygen (ROS) and nitrogen (RNS) species

These are commonly used generic terms to describe both free radical species and reactive non-radical molecules that can give rise to free radicals. Table 16 shows examples of important ROS and RNS. ROS and RNS are produced constantly in healthy cells at low concentrations when they perform essential functions.

Positive effects of FRs

- Free radicals stimulate cell growth, differentiation and signalling, e.g. sensing O_2 concentration.
- Free radicals induce protective enzymes.
- Cellular protection following the inflammatory response to injury and infection.
- NO plays a vital role in vasodilation.

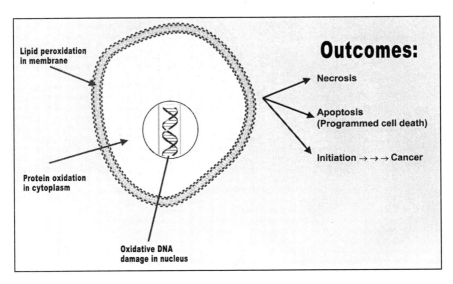

Figure 9 **Cellular reactive oxygen species overload.**

Negative effects of free radicals

- At higher concentrations cell membranes are oxidised and destabilised.

- Protein oxidation can cause structural damage and modulation of enzyme activity

- ROS damage to DNA can result in mutation. Figure 9 shows the main sites of ROS damage in the cell and the potential outcomes.

- Tissue injury and toxic insult can give rise to conditions of ROS overload which can swamp the body's endogenous protective system. Figure 10 shows how ROS are generated in response to injury or toxic insult.

Table 16 **Examples of important ROS and RNS**

ROS	RNS
Hydroxyl radical (OH$\cdot$) is the most reactive and attacks all biological molecules	Nitric oxide (NO$\cdot$) has a crucial role in vasodilation and Fe uptake
Superoxide ($O_2^-\cdot$) is usually the first FR to be formed during oxidative stress. It is converted to:	Peroxynitrite (ONOO$^-$) may initiate the process of lipid peroxidation in low density lipoprotein particles (LDL)
Hydrogen peroxide (H_2O_2) is much less active but can form OH$\cdot$ in the presence of Fe^{2+}	
Hypochlorous acid (HOCl, bleach) is produced by activated neutrophils in response to pathogen infection	

Figure 10

Tissue injury, oxidative stress and the effects of protective diets. Stages 1 and 2 are exacerbated by antioxidant-poor diets. Dietary tomatoes and their products can protect against oxidative stress by preventing and reducing ROS production at Stages 1 and 2.

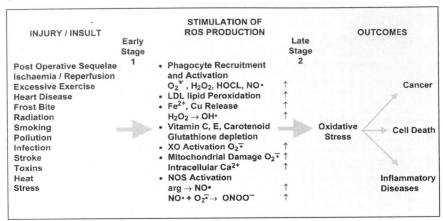

The body's antioxidant defence system

Preventative antioxidant proteins which sequester the toxic metals copper and iron are: transferrin (Fe), ferritin (Fe), caeruloplasmin (Cu), albumin (Cu). These help to prevent the formation of ROS.

Scavenging enzymes and antioxidants

Antioxidant enzymes

Superoxide dismutase (SOD)

$$2O_2^{-\bullet} + 2H^+ \rightarrow H_2O_2 + O_2$$

Catalase (CAT)

$$2H_2O_2 \rightarrow 2H_2O + O_2$$

232

Glutathione peroxidase (GPx)

$$ROOH + 2GSH \rightarrow ROH + H_2O + GSSG$$

Glutathione reductase (GR)

$$NADPH + H^+ + GSSG \rightarrow NADP^{\bullet} + 2GSH$$

Low molecular weight endogenous antioxidants (AO)

Glutathione, bilirubin and uric acid also provide protection from the damaging effects of ROS.

Is there a requirement for additional protection?

In the absence of adequate dietary protection, the body's AO defence system is not adequate for coping with large increases in ROS production, and damaging species may be transported to the nucleus where genetic damage could occur (Figure 9). The cell has evolved a sophisticated system of protection and repair to maintain the fidelity of the DNA which can sustain 10^6 damaging events per cell per day. Nevertheless, ROS overload can lead to genetic damage and cell transformation.

How and where are ROS generated?

Figure 11 shows the various sites at which ROS can be generated and where dietary AO can confer protection.

The role of ROS in heart disease

Cardiovascular disease is a major cause of death in the developed world before the age of 65, and its incidence is diet-related. ROS and RNS play a critical role in the initiation and progression of atherosclerosis, and many studies have shown dietary anti-

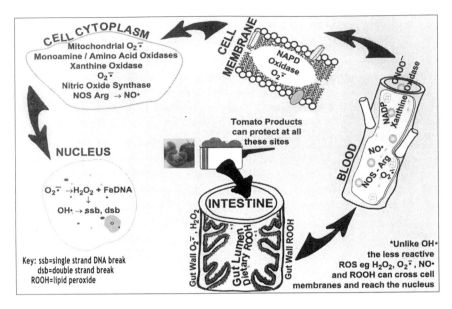

Figure 11 **ROS, antioxidants and vascular damage.**

oxidants to have a protective effect. Figure 12 shows how atherogenesis is initiated and how it progresses by the ROS/RNS mediated oxidation of LDL.

It is important to realise that oxidative damage occurs not on the blood vessel surface, but in the intima, in the space between the endothelium and the vascular smooth muscle cells (SMC). Native LDL enter the intima and undergo RNS/ROS attack to form oxidised LDL (oxoLDL) that stimulate the expression of adhesion molecules on the endothelial cells which sequester blood monocytes and prevent the exit of macrophages from the intima. Macrophages take up oxoLDL in an uncontrolled manner to form foam cells, which can release cytokines and stimulate SMC proliferation or undergo necrosis to release lipids and lysosomal enzymes into the intima. This results in a thickening of the vessel wall and ultimately plaque formation as a result of endothelial cell injury. Further oxidative damage to the plaque can lead to platelet aggregation and vessel blockage. Many studies in animals and humans indicate that tomato components can reduce the initiating reactions in atherogenesis which are driven by the oxidation of LDL.

How is the body's antioxidant defence integrated?

The metal binding proteins and the endogenous enzymes (SOD, CAT, GPx and GR) serve as a first line of defence in preventing the formation of ROS, or together with bilirubin and urate scavenge pre-formed ROS.

What happens to the ROS that evade the above system? Note that the above system has evolved to detoxify ROS/RNS in the aqueous compartment of the cell. There is no endogenous mechanism that can destroy oil-soluble radicals within the cell membrane, and a crucial problem is the high solubility of oxygen in lipid membranes which exacerbates lipid peroxidation.

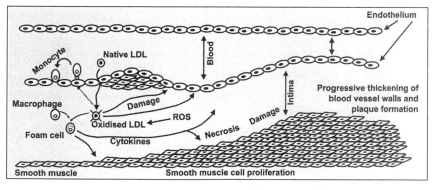

Figure 12 **ROS, antioxidants and vascular damage.**

235

Tomato-rich diets supply lycopene, β-carotene, and vitamin E which are oil-soluble and become incorporated into the LDL particles, where they act in a concerted manner to inhibit lipid peroxidation, to yield the relatively unreactive α-tocopherol radical (α-tocopherol˙) as an end product. Vitamin E is regenerated at the surface of the LDL by vitamin C and glutathione present in the aqueous environment, by an analogous mechanism to that shown in Figure 13.

The role of the tomato in healthy diets

We use the tomato here as a model because it contains high concentrations of lycopene and β-carotene in addition to the

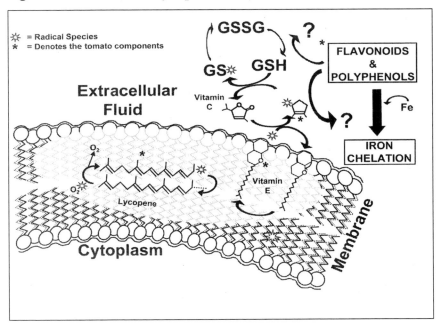

Figure 13 Biological regeneration of free radical scavengers.

important antioxidants found in other fruit and vegetables. The tomato is a major constituent in what is referred to as the Mediterranean Diet, which is purported to have considerable health benefits. Tomato provides the sole source of the red carotenoid lycopene, together with β-carotene which has many known health benefits, and the cooked products such as concentrated paste and pasta sauce which contain added vitamin E as a stabiliser.

Fresh tomatoes also contain a substantial amount of water-soluble antioxidants such as vitamin C, polyphenols and flavonoids. It is also a rich source of folic acid which may play a crucial role in the prevention of CVD and cancer, and is known to prevent neural tube defects in the developing foetus.

Why are tomato components of importance in human health?

Over 100 human diseases ranging from cancer and CVD to arthritis and Parkinson's disease involve oxidative stress and free radicals in their development. Antioxidant pigments and vitamins can scavenge these free radicals, reducing oxidative stress and the subsequent disease symptoms. The tomato provides a balanced mixture of both water-soluble and oil-soluble antioxidants, capable of protecting the cell membrane and its contents from free radical attack.

Role of dietary tomato components

It is the oil-soluble components that are vital in protecting the cell membrane against ROS mediated damage. Lycopene is able to detoxify superoxide by electron abstraction to form oxygen and a lycopene anion radical. This radical may then interact with vitamin E to regenerate lycopene and form α-tocopherol'. Regeneration of vitamin E can then take place on the surface of the membrane by hydrogen abstraction via ascorbate and glutathione. Although no direct evidence is currently available, the structure and reactivity of the tomato polyphenols and flavonoids would allow their potential involvement in radical scavenging and metal chelating functions (Figure 13).

Gap junction communication

Healthy cells communicate via small intercellular pores (gap junctions) through which small signal molecules can pass. Tumour cells have lost these pores and do not respond. However, initiated cells still respond via these pores and can be prevented from progressing to metaplastic cells by signals from their healthy neighbours.

β-Carotene has been shown to up regulate the synthesis of gap junction proteins via its role in retinoid formation. Lycopene, although not a retinoid, causes a slight increase in gap junction synthesis. Retinoids are important in cell growth and differentiation and are known to suppress the growth of some tumour cells.

Lycopene and β-carotene are non-polar carotenoids which do not interact with the polar phospholipid surface of the cell membrane. Results from our laboratory at JMU Liverpool indicate that lycopene can protect cells from oxidative DNA damage only at physiologically relevant concentrations (i.e. less than 1μM) [214]. Higher concentrations led to a progressive loss of protection and an associated increase in membrane permeability, and DNA damage. These results may have bearing on the previous ATBC and aborted CARET β-carotene intervention trials, where synthetic β-carotene was administered and blood levels were well above those normally attained from a healthy diet, and led to a 20% increase in the incidence of cancer in the carotenoid supplemented patients. It is possible that high concentrations of non-polar carotenoids may cause disruption of the membrane and allow ROS and their reactive products to target the nucleus.

Intervention studies in the US on the uptake, bioavailability and half-life of blood carotenoids, using healthy subjects on self-selected diets, have yielded useful data on lycopene. Lycopene repletion following a diet rich in pasta sauce reached approximately 1μM in the plasma. After seven days on a carotenoid-free diet, the lycopene levels had dropped to around 100nM. Under the same regime, β-carotene levels dropped from 200nM to 150nM. These interesting observations indicate that lycopene may possibly have an important role as a sacrificial antioxidant by virtue of its increased sensitivity to oxygen and ROS/RNS as compared to other carotenoids. On a more basic level, these studies have shown the importance of consuming cooked tomato products to optimise the uptake of lycopene.

Conclusions

All the single compound trials, whether they involved carotenoids or the antioxidant vitamins, tended to yield equivocal results. Attempts to design experiments to assess potential synergies have been fraught with difficulties, but have yielded more meaningful results. They have brought us closer to an understanding of how to optimise antioxidant protection by sensible dietary modification. The carotenoids, natural vitamin E, and vitamin C are now firmly established as protective dietary antioxidants with additional beneficial functions. Polyphenols and flavonoids are also gaining prominence and the protective role of folate is above dispute. All of these components are uniquely found in fresh and cooked tomatoes, which underlines why they are important in healthy diets, together with a wide range of fruit and vegetables.

Research over the past three decades has provided a scientific basis to support the common wisdom that diets rich in fruit and vegetables are beneficial to health. The protective role of antioxidant-rich diets in disease progression and ageing are beyond doubt, and advances in medicine over the past half century have resulted in a significant increase in lifespan in the developed world. The aged population has escaped the ravages of infectious diseases only to become prone to the long-term chronic ailments associated with oxidative stress such as CVD, arthritis and macular degeneration, as a result of inappropriate diets and lifestyles. Current research is now revealing the mechanisms behind all the old observational studies on diet and health.

REFERENCES

1. Lambe, W., *Additional reports on the effects of a peculiar regimen in cases of cancer, scrofula, consumption, asthma and other chronic diseases.* Mawman, 1815, London.

2. Banting, W., *Letter on Corpulence.* 3rd ed., 1864, London Harrison, 59 Pall Mall.

3. Hoffman, F., *Cancer and Diet.* 1937, Baltimore: The Williams and Wilkins Co.

4. Keys, A., *Mediterranean diet and public health: personal reflections.* American Journal of Clinical Nutrition, 1995. **61**(suppl): 1321S-1323S.

5. Wynder, E.L. and Gori, G.B., *Contribution of the environment to cancer incidence: an epidemiologic exercise.* Journal of the National Cancer Institute, 1977. **58**(4): 825-832.

6. Trichopoulou A, *et al.*, *Vegetable and fruit: the evidence in their favour and the public health perspective.* Int J Vitam Nutr Res , 2003. **73(2)**: 63-69.

7. Crawford, M.A., *The role of dietary fatty acids in biology: their place in the evolution of the human brain.* Nutrition Reviews, 1992. **50**(4): 3.

8. Grandinetti, A., *Prevalence of overweight and central adiposity is associated with percentage of indigenous ancestry among native Hawaiians.* International Journal of Obesity, 1999. **23**(7): 733.

9. Imazu, M., *Influence of type 2 diabetes mellitus on cardiovascular disease mortality: findings from the Hawaii-Los Angeles-Hiroshima study.* Diabetes Research and Clinical Practice, 2002. **57**(1): 61.

10. Simmons, D., *Polynesians: prone to obesity and Type 2 diabetes mellitus but not hyperinsulinaemia.* Diabetic Medicine, 2001. **18**(3): 193.

11. Cahill, G.F. Jr, and Owen, O.E., *Starvation and survival.* Trans Am Clin Climat Ass, 1967. **79**: 13-18.

12. Kark, R., Johnson, R. and Lewis, J., *Defects of pemmican as an emergency ration for infantry troops.* War Medicine, 1946. **8**: 345-352.

13. Stackpole, E., *The long arctic search: The narrative of Lieutenant Frederick Schwatka, USA, 1878-1880, seeking the records of the lost Franklin expedition.* Marine Historical Association, 1965.

14. Phinney, S., *Ketogenic diets and physical performance.* Nutrition & Metabolism, 2004. **1**(1): 2-2.

15. Annison, G., *Nutritional role of resistant starch: chemical structure vs physiological function.* Annual Review of Nutrition, 1994. **14**(1): 297.

16. Wolever, T.M., *Glycemic response to pasta: effect of surface area, degree of cooking, and protein enrichment.* Diabetes Care, 1986. **9**(4): 401.

17. Wolever, T., *Glycaemic index of 102 complex carbohydrate foods in patients with diabetes.* Nutrition Research, 1994. **14**(5): 651.

18. Haber, G., *et al.*, *Depletion and disruption of dietary fibre: effects on satiety, plasma-glucose, and serum-insulin.* Lancet, 1977. **310**(8040): 679.

19. Wegge, J.K., *et al.*, *Effect of diet and exercise intervention on inflammatory and adhesion molecules in postmenopausal women on hormone replacement therapy and at risk for coronary artery disease.* Metabolism, Clinical and Experimental, 2004. **53**(3): 377-81.

20. Defra, *Family Food in 2006. A National Statistics Publication.* 2006, Office of National Statistics.

21. Wang, G.-J., et al., *Brain dopamine and obesity.* Lancet, 2001. **357**(9253): 354.

22. Johnsson, P.M. and Kenny, P.J., *Dopamine D2 receptor s in addiction like reward dysfunction and compulsive eating in obese rats.* Nature Neuroscience, 2010. **13**: 635-641.

23. Stice, E., *et al.*, *Relation between obesity and blunted striatal response to food is moderated by TaqIA A1 allele.* Science, 2008. **322**(5900): 449.

24. Stice, E., *et al.*, *Reward circuitry responsivity to food predicts future increases in body mass: Moderating effects of DRD2 and DRD4.* NeuroImage, 2010. **50**(4): 1618-1625.

25. Gao, X., *Intake of added sugar and sugar-sweetened drink and serum uric acid concentration in US men and women.* Hypertension, 2007. **50**(2): 306.

26. Sanchez, A., *Role of sugars in human neutrophilic phagocytosis.* American Journal of Clinical Nutrition, 1973. **26**(11): 1180.

27. Nosadini, R. and Tonolo, G., *Blood glucose and lipid control as risk factors in the progression of renal damage in type 2 diabetes.* JN. Journal of Nephrology, 2003. **16** Suppl 7: S42-S47.

28. Gotto, A.M., *Triglyceride: the forgotten risk factor.* Circulation, 1998. **97**(11): 1027.

29. Parks, E.J., *Carbohydrate-induced hypertriacylglycerolemia: historical perspective and review of biological mechanisms.* American Journal of Clinical Nutrition, 2000. **71**(2): 412.

30. Lindsay, R. and Howard, B., *Cardiovascular risk associated with the metabolic syndrome.* Current Diabetes Reports, 2004. **4**(1): 63-68.

31. Sowers, J.R., *Update on the cardiometabolic syndrome.* Clinical Cornerstone, 2001. **4**(2): 17-23.

32. Aronson, D., *Association between fasting glucose and C-reactive protein in middle-aged subjects.* Diabetic Medicine, 2004. **21**(1): 39.

33. Bonnefont-Rousselot, D., *Glucose and reactive oxygen species.* Current Opinion in Clinical Nutrition and Metabolic Care, 2002. **5**(5): 561.

34. Andreadis, A.A., *Oxidative and nitrosative events in asthma.* Free Radical Biology & Medicine, 2003. **35**(3): 213.

35. Behrend, L., *Reactive oxygen species in oncogenic transformation.* Biochemical Society Transactions, 2003. **31**: 1441.

36. Hadjigogos, K., *The role of free radicals in the pathogenesis of rheumatoid arthritis.* Panminerva Med., 2003. **45**(1): 7-13.

37. McGeer, E.G., *Inflammatory processes in Alzheimer's disease.* Progress in Neuro-psychopharmacology & Biological Psychiatry, 2003. **27**(5): 741.

38. Warburg, O., *On the origin of cancer cells.* Science, 1956. **123**(3191): 309.

39. Higginbotham, S., *Dietary glycemic load and risk of colorectal cancer in the Women's Health Study.* Journal of the National Cancer Institute, 2004. **96**(3): 229.

40. Brand-Miller, J.C., *Glycemic load and chronic disease.* Nutrition Reviews, 2003. **61**: S49.

41. Seyfried, T.N., *Role of glucose and ketone bodies in the metabolic control of experimental brain cancer.* British Journal of Cancer, 2003. **89**(7): 1375.

42. Renehan, A.G., *Insulin-like growth factor (IGF)-I, IGF binding protein-3, and cancer risk: systematic review and meta-regression analysis.* Lancet, 2004. **363**(9418): 1346.

43. van Halteren, H., Bongaerts, G. and Wagener, D., *Cancer cachexia: what is known about its etiology and what should be the current treatment approach?* Anticancer Res Nov-Dec, 2003. **23**(6D): 5111-5115.

44. Ayre, S.G., Perez Garcia y Bellon, D. and Garcia, D.P., *Neoadjuvant low-dose chemotherapy with insulin in breast carcinomas.* European Journal of Cancer, 1990. **26**(11-12): 1262-1263.

45. Alabaster, O., *Metabolic modification by insulin enhances methotrexate cytotoxicity in MCF-7 human breast cancer cells.* European Journal of Cancer & Clinical Oncology, 1981. **17**(11): 1223.

46. Ludwig, D.S., *Diet and development of the insulin resistance syndrome.* Asia Pacific Journal of Clinical Nutrition, 2003. **12** Suppl: S4-S4.

47. Pradeepa, R. and Mohan, V., *The changing scenario of the diabetes epidemic: implications for India.* Indian Journal of Medical Research, 2002. **116**: 121-132.

48. WHO, *Technical report 916: Diet, nutrition and the prevention of chronic disease*, WHO, Editor. 2003: Geneva

49. Davoli, E., *Serum methanol concentrations in rats and in men after a single dose of aspartame.* Food and Chemical Toxicology, 1986. **24**(3): 187.

50. Monte, W.C., *Aspartame: methanol and the public health.* Journal of Applied Nutrition, 1984. **36**(1): 42-54.

51. Posner, H.S., *Biohazards of methanol in proposed new uses.* Journal of Toxicology and Environmental Health. Part B, 1975. **1**(1): 153.

245

52. He, J.L., Jin, L.F. and Jin, H.Y., *Detection of cytogenetic effects in peripheral lymphocytes of students exposed to formaldehyde with cytokinesis-blocked micronucleus assay.* Biomedical Environmental Science, 1998. **11**(1): 87-92.

53. Liu, K.S., *Irritant effects of formaldehyde exposure in mobile homes.* Environmental Health Perspectives, 1991. **94**: 91.

54. Main, D.M., *Health effects of low-level exposure to formaldehyde.* Journal of Occupational and Environmental Medicine, 1983. **25**(12): 896.

55. Adam, A., *et al.*, *Impact of whole wheat flour and its milling fractions on the cecal fermentations and the plasma and liver lipids in rats.* Journal of Agricultural and Food Chemistry, 2002. **50**(22): 6557.

56. Lang, R. and Jebb, S., *Who consumes whole grains, and how much?* Proceedings of the Nutrition Society, 2003. **62**(01): 123.

57. Gannon, M. and Nuttall, F., *Protein and diabetes*, in American Diabetes Association Guide to Medical Nutrition Therapy for Diabetes. 1999: Alexandria. 107-25.

58. Conn, J.W., *The glycemic response to isoglucogenic quantities of protein and carbohydrate.* Journal of Clinical Investigation, 1936. **15**(6): 665.

59. Nuttall, P.F. and Gannon, M., *Plasma glucose and insulin response to macronutrients in nondiabetics and NIDDM subjects.* Diabetes Care, 1991. **14**: 824-38.

60. Westphal, S.A., *Metabolic response to glucose ingested with various amounts of protein.* American Journal of Clinical Nutrition, 1990. **52**(2): 267.

61. Dwyer, J.T., *Diet, indicators of kidney disease, and later mortality among older persons in the NHANES I Epidemiologic Follow-Up Study.* American Journal of Public Health, 1994. **84**(8): 1299.

62. Enig, M., *Saturated fats and the kidneys.* Wise Traditions, 2000. **1**(3): 49.

63. Chandra, R.K., *Nutrition and the immune system from birth to old age.* European Journal of Clinical Nutrition, 2002. **56** Suppl 3: S73-S76.

64. Keusch, G.T., *The history of nutrition: malnutrition, infection and immunity.* Journal of Nutrition, 2003. **133**(1): 336S.

65. Webb, J., Kiess, M. and Chan-Yan, C., *Malnutrition and the heart.* . CMAJ, 1986. **135**(7): 753-758.

66. Pichard, C., *et al.*, *Recombinant human growth hormone in chronic and acute respiratory insufficiency.* Horm Res, 1996. **46**(4-5): 222-229.

67. Ginty, F., *Dietary protein and bone health.* Proceedings of the Nutrition Society, 2003. **62**(04): 867.

68. Feskanich, D., *Protein consumption and bone fractures in women.* American Journal of Epidemiology, 1996. **143**(5): 472.

69. Dawson-Hughes, B., *Effect of dietary protein supplements on calcium excretion in healthy older men and women.* Journal of Clinical Endocrinology and Metabolism, 2004. **89**(3): 1169.

70. Tucker, K.L., *The acid-base hypothesis: diet and bone in the Framingham Osteoporosis Study.* European Journal of Nutrition, 2001. **40**(5): 231.

71. Cumming, R.G., *Case-control study of risk factors for hip fractures in the elderly.* American Journal of Epidemiology, 1994. **139**(5): 493.

72. De Stefani, E., *Meat intake, heterocyclic amines, and risk of breast cancer: a case-control study in Uruguay.* Cancer Epidemiology, Biomarkers & Prevention, 1997. **6**(8): 573.

247

73. Terry, P.D., *Dietary intake of heterocyclic amines and cancers of the esophagus and gastric cardia.* Cancer Epidemiology, Biomarkers & Prevention, 2003. **12**(9): 940.

74. Farnsworth, E., *Effect of a high-protein, energy-restricted diet on body composition, glycemic control, and lipid concentrations in overweight and obese hyperinsulinemic men and women.* American Journal of Clinical Nutrition, 2003. **78**(1): 31.

75. Hu, F.B., Stamfer, M.J. and Manson, J.E. *Dietary protein and the risk of heart disease in women.* Am J Clin Nutr 1999, **70**: 221-227.

76. Zhang, X., *et al., Soy food consumption is associated with lower risk of coronary heart disease in Chinese women.* Journal of Nutrition, 2003. **133**(9): 2874.

77. Anderson, J.W., Johnstone, B.M. and Cook-Newell, M.E., *Meta-analysis of the effects of soy protein intake on serum lipids.* New England Journal of Medicine, 1995. **333**(5): 276.

78. Ashton, E.L., *Effect of meat replacement by tofu on CHD risk factors including copper induced LDL oxidation.* Journal of the American College of Nutrition, 2000. **19**(6): 761.

79. Hasler, C.M., *The cardiovascular effects of soy products.* Journal of Cardiovascular Nursing, 2002. **16**(4): 50.

80. Messina, M., *Gaining insight into the health effects of soy but a long way still to go: commentary on the fourth International Symposium on the Role of Soy in Preventing and Treating Chronic Disease.* Journal of Nutrition, 2002. **132**(3): 547S.

81. Persaud, D.R., *Bovine serum albumin and insulin-dependent diabetes mellitus: is cow's milk still a possible toxicological causative agent of diabetes?* Food and Chemical Toxicology, 2004. **42**(5): 707.

82. de Lemos, M., *Effects of soy phytoestrogens genistein and daidzein on breast cancer growth.* Ann Pharmacother, 2001. **35**: 1118-1121.

83. Patisaul, H. and Jefferson, W., *The pros and cons of phytoestrogens.* Front Neuroendocrinol, 2010. **31**(4): 400-419.

84. Velentzis, L.S., *Do phytoestrogens reduce the risk of breast cancer and breast cancer recurrence? What clinicians need to know.* European Journal of Cancer, 2008. **44**(13): 1799.

85. Roebuck, B.D., *Enhancement of pancreatic carcinogenesis by raw soy protein isolate: quantitative rat model and nutritional considerations.* Adv Exp Med Biol, 1986. **199**: 91-107.

86. Schmitt, E., *Genotoxic activity of four metabolites of the soy isoflavone daidzein.* Mutation Research – Genetic Toxicology and Environmental Mutagenesis, 2003. **542**(1-2): 43.

87. Doerge, D.R., *Inactivation of thyroid peroxidase by soy isoflavones, in vitro and in vivo.* Journal of Chromatography, 2002. **777**(1-2): 269.

88. Knekt, P., *et al.*, *Risk of colorectal and other gastro-intestinal cancers after exposure to nitrate, nitrite and N-nitroso compounds: a follow-up study.* International Journal of Cancer, 1999. **80**(6): 852.

89. Adamson, R.H. and Thorgeirsson, U.P., *Carcinogens in foods: heterocyclic amines and cancer and heart disease.* Adv Exp Med Biol, 1995. **369**: 211-220.

90. Chenoweth, W., *Influence of dietary cholesterol and fat on serum lipids in men.* Journal of Nutrition, 1981. **111**(12): 2069.

91. Sacks, F.M., *Lack of an effect of dietary saturated fat and cholesterol on blood pressure in normotensives.* Hypertension, 1984. **6**(2): 193.

92. Addis, P., Food and Nutrition News, 1990. **62**(2): 7-10.

93. Holub, D.J., *Omega-3 fatty acids from fish oils and cardiovascular disease.* Molecular and Cellular Biochemistry, 2004. **263**(1): 217.

94. Menotti, A., *Food intake patterns and 25-year mortality from coronary heart disease: cross-cultural correlations in the Seven Countries Study.* European Journal of Epidemiology, 1999. **15**(6): 507.

95. Simon, J.A., *Serum fatty acids and the risk of coronary heart disease.* American Journal of Epidemiology, 1995. **142**(5): 469.

96. Salmeron, J., *Dietary fat intake and risk of type 2 diabetes in women.* American Journal of Clinical Nutrition, 2001. **73**(6): 1019.

97. de Roos, N., Schouten, E. and Katan, M., *Trans fatty acids, HDL-cholesterol, and cardiovascular disease. Effects of dietary changes on vascular reactivity.* Eur J Med Res, 2003. **20**(8): 355-357.

98. Lichtenstein, A.H., *Influence of hydrogenated fat and butter on CVD risk factors: remnant-like particles, glucose and insulin, blood pressure and C-reactive protein.* Atherosclerosis, 2003. **171**(1): 97.

99. Felton, C.V., *Dietary polyunsaturated fatty acids and composition of human aortic plaques.* Lancet, 1994. **344**(8931): 1195.

100. Elson, C.E., *The influence of dietary unsaturated cis and trans and saturated fatty acids on tissue lipids of swine.* Atherosclerosis, 1981. **40**(2): 115.

101. Kohlmeier, L., *Adipose tissue trans fatty acids and breast cancer in the European Community Multicenter Study on Antioxidants, Myocardial Infarction, and Breast Cancer.* Cancer Epidemiology, Biomarkers & Prevention, 1997. **6**(9): 705.

102. Wolk, A., *Insulin-like growth factor 1 and prostate cancer risk: a population-based, case-control study.* Journal of the National Cancer Institute, 1998. **90**(12): 911.

103. Smith-Warner, S., *Types of dietary fat and breast cancer: a pooled analysis of cohort studies.* International Journal of Cancer, 2001. **92**(5): 767.

104. Mann, G.V., *Metabolic consequences of dietary trans fatty acids.* Lancet, 1994. **343**(8908): 1268.

105. Enig, M.G., Munn, R.J. and Keeney, M., *Dietary fat and cancer trends - a critique.* Federation Proceedings, 1978. **37**(9): 2215-2220.

106. Stoll, B.A., *Breast cancer and the western diet: role of fatty acids and antioxidant vitamins.* European Journal of Cancer, 1998. **34**: 1852.

107. Aro, A., *Epidemiology of trans fatty acids and coronary heart disease in Europe.* Nutrition Metabolism and Cardiovascular Diseases, 1998. **8**(6): 402-407.

108. Koletzko, B., *Metabolic aspects of trans fatty acids.* Clinical Nutrition, 1997. **16**(5): 229.

109. Larqué, E., *Dietary trans fatty acids affect docosahexaenoic acid concentrations in plasma and liver but not brain of pregnant and fetal rats.* Pediatric Research, 2000. **47**(2): 278.

110. Koletzko, B., *Potential adverse effects of trans fatty acids in infants and children.* European Journal of Medical Research, 1995. **1**(2): 123-125.

111. Rabinowitz, D., *et al., Patterns of hormonal release after glucose, protein, and glucose plus protein.* Lancet, 1966. **2**(7461): 454-456.

251

112. Strandvik, B., *et al.*, *Is the relatively low intake of omega-3 fatty acids in Western diet contributing to the obesity epidemics?* Lipid Tech, 2008. **20**(3): 49-72.

113. Shaper, A.G., *Cardiovascular studies in the Samburu tribe of Northern Kenya.* American Heart Journal, 1962. **63**(4): 437.

114. UN, *Food intake data from Food and Agriculture Organization of the United Nations, Statistical Database. CHD mortality data.*, World Health Statistics Annual. 1999.

115. Kritchevsky, D., *Dietary protein, cholesterol and atherosclerosis: a review of the early history.* Journal of Nutrition, 1995. **125**(3 Suppl): 589S.

116. Steiner, A. and Kendall, F.E., *Atherosclerosis and arteriosclerosis in dogs following ingestion of cholesterol and thiouracil.* Archives of Pathology, 1946. **42**: 433-444.

117. Williams, C.W., Proceedings of the Nutrition Society, 1997. **56**: 679-692.

118. Calle, E.E., Rodriguez, C., Walker-Thurmond, B. and Thun, M.J., *Overweight, obesity, and mortality from cancer in a prospectively studied cohort of U.S. adults.* N Engl J Med, 2003. **348**: 1625-1638.

119. Muskiet, F.A.J., *Is docosahexaenoic acid (DHA) essential? Lessons from DHA status regulation, our ancient diet, epidemiology and randomized controlled trials.* Journal of Nutrition, 2004. **134**(1): 183.

120. Beisiegel, U., *Lipoprotein (a) in the arterial wall.* European Heart Journal, 1990. **11**(suppl E): 174.

121. Hooper, L., *et al.*, *Dietary fat intake and prevention of cardiovascular disease: systematic review.* Quality & Safety in Health Care, 2001. **322**(7289): 757.

252

122. Sanders, T.A.B., *et al.*, *Influence of fatty acid chain length and cis/trans isomerization on postprandial lipemia and factor VII in healthy subjects (postprandial lipids and factor VII).* Atherosclerosis, 2000. **149**(2): 413-420.

123. Mensink, R.P., *et al.*, *Effects of dietary fatty acids and carbohydrates on the ratio of serum total to HDL cholesterol and on serum lipids and apolipoproteins: a meta-analysis of 60 controlled trials.* American Journal of Clinical Nutrition, 2003. **77**(5): 1146-1155.

124. Berglund, L., *et al.*, *HDL-subpopulation patterns in response to reductions in dietary total and saturated fat intakes in healthy subjects.* American Journal of Clinical Nutrition, 1999. **70**(6): 992-1000.

125. Mensink, R.P., *Effect of dietary fatty acids on serum lipids and lipoproteins. A meta-analysis of 27 trials.* Arteriosclerosis, Thrombosis, and Vascular Biology, 1992. **12**(8): 911.

126. Tavvintharan, S. and Kashyap, M., *The benefits of niacin in atherosclerosis.* Curr Atheroscler Rep, 2001. **3**(1): 74-82.

127. Ridker, P.M., *Novel risk factors for systemic atherosclerosis: a comparison of C-reactive protein, fibrinogen, homocysteine, lipoprotein (a), and standard cholesterol screening as predictors of peripheral arterial disease.* JAMA, 2001. **285**(19): 2481.

128. Stanley, J., *Effects of dietary fatty acids on the ratio of total to HDL cholesterol.* Lipid Tech, 2004. **16**(9): 206-208.

129. Kelly, F.D., *et al.*, *Short-term diets enriched in stearic or palmitic acids do not alter plasma lipids, platelet aggregation or platelet activation status.* European Journal of Clinical Nutrition, 2002. **56**(6): 490.

130. Sanchez-Muniz, F.J., *Dietary fat saturation affects apolipoprotein AII levels and HDL composition in postmenopausal women.* Journal of Nutrition, 2002. **132**(1): 50.

131. Jeppesen, J., *Effects of low-fat, high-carbohydrate diets on risk factors for ischemic heart disease in postmenopausal women.* American Journal of Clinical Nutrition, 1997. **65**(4): 1027.

132. Kris-Etherton, P.M., *Monounsaturated fatty acids and risk of cardiovascular disease.* Circulation, 1999. **100**(11): 1253.

133. Liu, S., *et al.*, *A prospective study of dietary glycemic load, carbohydrate intake, and risk of coronary heart disease in US women.* American Journal of Clinical Nutrition, 2000. **71**(6): 1455.

134. Westman, E.C., *Is dietary carbohydrate essential for human nutrition?* American Journal of Clinical Nutrition, 2002. **75**(5): 951.

135. Abbasi, F., *et al.*, *High carbohydrate diets, triglyceride-rich lipoproteins, and coronary heart disease risk.* American Journal of Cardiology, 2000. **85**(1): 45.

136. Ellison, L.F., *Low serum cholesterol concentration and risk of suicide.* Epidemiology, 2001. **12**(2): 168.

137. Ridker, P.M., *et al.*, *C-reactive protein and other markers of inflammation in the prediction of cardiovascular disease in women.* New England Journal of Medicine, 2000. **23**(342(12)): 836-843.

138. Harjai, K.J., *Potential new cardiovascular risk factors: left ventricular hypertrophy, homocysteine, lipoprotein (a), triglycerides, oxidative stress, and fibrinogen.* Annals of Internal Medicine, 1999. **131**(5): 376.

139. Oh, J., *et al.*, *Genetic Determinants of Statin Intolerance.* Lipids in Health and Disease, 2007. **6**(7).

140. Lilja, J.J., Neuvonen, M., and Neuvonen, P.J., *Effects of regular consumption of grapefruit juice on the pharmacokinetics of simvastatin.* British Journal of Clinical Pharmacology, 2004. **58**(1): 56.

141. Stephensen, C.B., *Vitamin A, infection and immune function.* Annual Review of Nutrition, 2001. **21**(1): 167.

142. D'souza, R. and D'souza, R., *Vitamin A for the treatment of children with measles–a systematic review.* Journal of Tropical Pediatrics, 2002. **48**(6): 323.

143. Zhang, L.X., *Carotenoids enhance gap junctional communication and inhibit lipid peroxidation in C3H/10T1/2 cells: relationship to their cancer chemopreventive action.* Carcinogenesis, 1991. **12**(11): 2109.

144. Kaul, L., *et al., The role of diet in prostate cancer.* Nutr Cancer, 1987. **9**(2-3): 123-128.

145. Ziegler, E.E., Present Knowledge in Nutrition. 1996.

146. Lopez, R., Schwartz, J., and Cooperman, J., *Riboflavin deficiency in an adolescent population in New York City.* American Journal of Clinical Nutrition, 1980. **33**(6): 1283.

147. Schmitt-Graff, A. and Scheulen, M.E., *Prevention of adriamycin cardiotoxicity by niacin, isocitrate or N-acetyl-cysteine in mice. A morphological study.* Pathology, Research and Practice, 1986. **181**(2): 168-174.

148. Malik, S. and Kashyap, M., *Niacin, lipids, and heart disease.* Curr Cardiol Rep, 2003. **5**(6): 470-6.

149. Binaghi, P., *et al., Evaluation of the cholesterol-lowering effectiveness of pantethine in women in perimenopausal age.* Minerva Medica, 1990. **81**(6): 475-479.

150. Zhdanova, I.V., *et al., Sleep-inducing effects of low doses of melatonin ingested in the evening.* Clinical Pharmacology & Therapeutics, 1995. **57**(5): 552.

151. Tanne, D., *Prospective study of serum homocysteine and risk of ischemic stroke among patients with preexisting coronary heart disease.* Stroke, 2003. **34**(3): 632.

152. Morris, M.S., *Homocysteine and Alzheimer's disease.* Lancet Neurology, 2003. **2**(7): 425.

153. Trakatellis, A., *Pyridoxine deficiency: new approaches in immunosuppression and chemotherapy.* Postgraduate Medical Journal, 1997. **73**(864): 617.

154. Spellacy, W.N., Buhi, W.C. and Birk, S.A., *Vitamin B6 treatment of gestational diabetes mellitus: studies of blood glucose and plasma insulin.* American Journal of Obstetrics and Gynecology, 1977. **127**(6): 599-602.

155. Mahajan, M.K. and Singh, V., *Assessment of efficacy of pyridoxine in control of radiation induced sickness.* Journal of the Indian Medical Association, 1998. **96**(3): 82-83.

156. Shultz, T., *et al.*, *Effect of pyridoxine and pyridoxal on the in vitro growth of human malignant melanoma.* Anticancer Res. Nov-Dec, 1988. **8**(6): 1313-8.

157. Ellis, F. and Nasser, S., *A pilot study of vitamin B12 in the treatment of tiredness.* British Journal of Nutrition, 1973. **30**(02): 277.

158. Lapp, C. and Cheney, P., *The rationale for using high-dose cobalamin (vitamin B12).* CFIDS Chronicle Physicians' Forum, 1993 (Fall): 19–20.

159. Cathcart, R.r., *The vitamin C treatment of allergy and the normally unprimed state of antibodies.* Med Hypotheses, 1986. **21**(3): 307-21.

160. Ellender, G. and Gazelakis, T., *Growth and bone remodelling in a scorbutic rat model.* Australian Dental Journal, 1996. **41**(2): 97.

161. Chak, C.W., *No change in bone-specific alkaline phosphatase activities in cultured rat osteoblastic cells under L-ascorbate and β-glycerophosphate-induced mineralization.* Cell Biology International, 1995. **19**(12): 979.

162. Pointillart, A., *Vitamin C supplementation does not modify bone mineral content or mineral absorption in growing pigs.* Journal of Nutrition, 1997. **127**(8): 1514.

163. Webb, R., *Vitamin C. Give a boost to your immune system.* Diabetes Forecast, 2004. **57**(1): 17-9.

164. Birlouez-Aragon, I. and Tessier, F., *Antioxidant vitamins and degenerative pathologies. A review of vitamin C.* J Nutr Health Aging, 2003. **7**(2): 103-9.

165. Abdel-Wahab, Y.H.A., *et al.*, *Vitamin C supplementation decreases insulin glycation and improves glucose homeostasis in obese hyperglycemic (ob/ob) mice.* Metabolism, Clinical and Experimental, 2002. **51**(4): 514.

166. Eriksson, J. and Kohvakka, A., *Magnesium and ascorbic acid supplementation in diabetes mellitus.* Ann Nutr Metab, 1995. **39**(4): 217-23.

167. Turley, S.D., West, C.E. and Horton, B.J., *The role of ascorbic acid in the regulation of cholesterol metabolism and in the pathogenesis of atherosclerosis.* Atherosclerosis, 1976. **24**(1-2): 1.

168. Lynch, S.M., Gaziano, J.M. and Frei, B., *Ascorbic acid and atherosclerotic cardiovascular disease.* Sub-cellular Biochemistry, 1996. **25**: 331-367.

169. Ellis, G.R., *Acute effects of vitamin C on platelet responsiveness to nitric oxide donors and endothelial function in patients with chronic heart failure.* Journal of Cardiovascular Pharmacology, 2001. **37**(5): 564.

170. Head, K.A., *Ascorbic acid in the prevention and treatment of cancer.* Alternative Medicine Review, 1998. **3**(3): 174-186.

171. Jacob, R.A., *Vitamin C function and status in chronic disease.* Nutrition in Clinical Care, 2002. **5**(2): 66.

172. Fletcher, A.E., Breeze, E. and Shetty, P.S., *Antioxidant vitamins and mortality in older persons: findings from the nutrition add-on study to the Medical Research Council Trial of Assessment and Management of Older People in the Community.* American Journal of Clinical Nutrition, 2003. **78**(5): 999.

173. Kurl, S., *et al.*, *Plasma vitamin C modifies the association between hypertension and risk of stroke.* Stroke, 2002. **33**(6): 1568.

174. Wang, X. and Studzinski, G.P., *Kinase suppressor of RAS (KSR) amplifies the differentiation signal provided by low concentrations 1, 25-dihydroxyvitamin D3.* Journal of Cellular Physiology, 2004. **198**(3): 333.

175. Vasu, P., *Effect of vitamin D analog (1 HydroxyY D5) immunoconjugated to Her-2 antibody on breast cancer.* International Journal of Cancer, 2004. **108**: 922.

176. Christensen, G.L., *Sequential versus combined treatment of human breast cancer cells with antiestrogens and the vitamin D analogue EB1089 and evaluation of predictive markers for vitamin D treatment.* Breast Cancer Research and Treatment, 2004. **85**(1): 53.

177. Stewart, L. and Weigel, N., *Vitamin D and prostate cancer.* Experimental Biology and Medicine, 2004. **229**(4): 277-284.

178. Traber, M., *Vitamin E*, in Modern Nutrition in Health and Disease, Shils, M.E., *et al.*, Editors. 1999, Williams & Wilkins: Baltimore. 347-362.

179. Evans, H. and Bishop, K., *On the existence of a hitherto unrecognized dietary factor essential for reproduction.* Science, 1922. **56**(1458): 650.

180. Mueller-Cunningham, W.M., Quintana, R. and Kasim-Karakas, S.E., *An ad libitum, very low-fat diet results in weight loss and*

changes in nutrient intakes in postmenopausal women. Journal of the American Dietetic Association, 2003. **103**(12): 1600.

181. Jialal, I. and Fuller, C.J., *Effect of vitamin E, vitamin C and beta-carotene on LDL oxidation and atherosclerosis.* Canadian Journal of Cardiology, 1995. **11** Suppl G: 97G-103G.

182. Kartal, O.N., Negis, Y. and Aytan, N., *Molecular mechanisms of cholesterol or homocysteine effect in the development of atherosclerosis. Role of vitamin E.* Biofactors, 2003. **19**(1-2): 63-70.

183. Antoniades, C., *et al., Oxidative stress, antioxidant vitamins, and atherosclerosis.* Herz, 2003. **28**(7): 628.

184. Kinlay, S., *Long-term effect of combined vitamins E and C on coronary and peripheral endothelial function.* Journal of the American College of Cardiology, 2004. **43**(4): 629.

185. Stampfer, M.J., *et al., Vitamin E consumption and the risk of coronary heart disease in women.* New England Journal of Medicine, 1993. **328**(20): 1444.

186. Yusuf, S., *et al., Vitamin E supplementation and cardiovascular events in high-risk patients. The Heart Outcomes Prevention Evaluation Study Investigators.* New England Journal of Medicine, 2000. **342**(3): 154-160.

187. Chow, C.K., *Dietary vitamin E and selenium and toxicity of nitrite and nitrate.* Toxicology, 2002. **180**(2): 195.

188. Weitberg, A.B. and Corvese, D., *Effect of vitamin E and beta-carotene on DNA strand breakage induced by tobacco-specific nitrosamines and stimulated human phagocytes.* Journal of Experimental & Clinical Cancer Research, 1997. **16**(1): 11-14.

189. Bostick, R.M., *et al., Reduced risk of colon cancer with high intake of vitamin E: the Iowa Women's Health Study.* Cancer Research, 1993. **53**(18): 4230.

190. Curl, W.W., *Aging and exercise: Are they compatible in women?* Clinical Orthopaedics and Related Research, 2000. **372**: 151.

191. Paffenbarger, R.S.J., *et al.*, *Physical activity, all-cause mortality, and longevity of college alumni.* New England Journal of Medicine, 1986. **314**(10): 605.

192. Wu, K., *A prospective study on supplemental vitamin e intake and risk of colon cancer in women and men.* Cancer Epidemiology, Biomarkers & Prevention, 2002. **11**(11): 1298.

193. Graham, S., *et al.*, *Diet in the epidemiology of postmenopausal breast cancer in the New York State Cohort.* American Journal of Epidemiology, 1992. **136**(11): 1327.

194. McNeil, J.J., *Vitamin E supplementation and cataract: randomized controlled trial.* Ophthalmology, 2004. **111**(1): 75.

195. Teikari, J.M., *Incidence of cataract operations in Finnish male smokers unaffected by alpha tocopherol or beta carotene supplements.* Journal of Epidemiology and Community Health, 1998. **52**(7): 468.

196. Meydani, S., *et al.*, *Assessment of the safety of supplementation with different amounts of vitamin E in healthy older adults.* American Journal of Clinical Nutrition, 1998. **68**(2): 311.

197. Hensley, K., *et al.*, *New perspectives on vitamin E:[gamma]-tocopherol and carboxyethylhydroxychroman metabolites in biology and medicine.* Free Radical Biology & Medicine, 2004. **36**(1): 1.

198. Wagner, K. and Isnardy, B., *New Insights into Tocopherol Research with Emphasis on Gamma Tocopherol and Delta Tocopherol.* Lipid Technology., 2006. **18**(2): 36-40.

199. Mock, D., *Biotin*, in Modern Nutrition in Health and Disease, M. Shils, *et al.*, Editors. 1999, Williams and Wilkins: Baltimore. 459–66.

200. Truswell, A.S., *ABC of nutrition. Measuring nutrition.* Quality & Safety in Health Care, 1985. **291**(6504): 1258.

201. Green, N.S., *Folic acid supplementation and prevention of birth defects.* Journal of Nutrition, 2002. **132**(8): 2356S.

202. Wald, N., *Prevention of neural tube defects: results of the Medical Research Council Vitamin Study.* Lancet, 1991. **338**(8760): 131.

203. Lee, B.J., *Folic acid and vitamin B12 are more effective than vitamin B6 in lowering fasting plasma homocysteine concentration in patients with coronary artery disease.* European Journal of Clinical Nutrition, 2004. **58**(3): 481.

204. Giovannucci, E., *et al.*, *Folate, methionine, and alcohol intake and risk of colorectal adenoma.* Journal of the National Cancer Institute, 1993. **85**(11): 875.

205. Lashner, B.A., *et al.*, *Effect of folate supplementation on the incidence of dysplasia and cancer in chronic ulcerative colitis. A case-control study.* Gastroenterology, 1989. **97**(2): 255-259.

206. Zhang, S., *et al.*, *A prospective study of folate intake and the risk of breast cancer.* JAMA, 1999. **281**(17): 1632.

207. Merck, *The Merck Manual®.* 1997, NJ: Merck Research Laboratories: Whitehouse Station.

208. Krinsky, N.I., *Effects of carotenoids in cellular and animal systems.* American Journal of Clinical Nutrition, 1991. **53**(1): 238S.

209. Bertram, J.S., *Structure-activity relationships among various retinoids and their ability to inhibit neoplastic transformation and to increase cell adhesion in the C3H/10T1/2 CL8 cell line.* Cancer Research, 1980. **40**(9): 3141-3146.

210. Peroccoa, P., *et al.*, *[beta]-Carotene as enhancer of cell transforming activity of powerful carcinogens and cigarette-*

261

smoke condensate on BALB/c 3T3 cells in vitro. Mutation Research – Genetic Toxicology and Environmental Mutagenesis, 1999. **440**(1): 83.

211. Collins, A.R., *Carotenoids and genomic stability.* Mutation Research – Genetic Toxicology and Environmental Mutagenesis, 2001. **475**(1-2): 21.

212. Burton, G.W., *Antioxidant action of carotenoids.* Journal of Nutrition, 1989. **119**(1): 109-111.

213. Heinonen, O. and Albanes, D., *The effect of vitamin E and beta carotene on the incidence of lung cancer and other cancers in male smokers.* New England Journal of Medicine, 1994. **330**: 1029.

214. Lowe, G., *et al.*, *Lycopene and β-carotene protect against oxidative damage in HT29 cells at low concentrations but rapidly lose this capacity at higher doses.* Free Radical Research, 1999. **30**(2): 141.

215. Giovannucci, E., *Intake of carotenoids and retino in relation to risk of prostate cancer.* Journal of the National Cancer Institute, 1995. **87**(23): 1767.

216. Hanley, D.Q., *Tomatoes, Oranges, Pasta and Soybeans Studied as Cancer Fighters.* AP, 1997.

217. Kumpulainen, J. and Salonen, J., *Natural Antioxidants and Food Quality in Atherosclerosis and Cancer Prevention*, Royal Society of Chemistry Information. 1996.

218. Mares-Perlman, J.A., *Serum antioxidants and age-related macular degeneration in a population-based case-control study.* Archives of Ophthalmology, 1995. **113**(12): 1518.

219. Aviram, M., *Lycopene and Atherosclerosis*, in Tomato Power! Lycopene: The Miracle Nutrient That Can Prevent Aging, Heart Disease and Cancer, F.J. Scheer, Editor. 1999, Technion-Israel

Institute of Technology and Advanced Research Press: Hauppauge, N.Y.

220. Gu, D., *et al.*, *Effect of potassium supplementation on blood pressure in Chinese: a randomized, placebo-controlled trial.* Journal of Hypertension, 2001. **19**(7): 1325.

221. Whelton, P.K., *et al.*, *Effects of oral potassium on blood pressure: meta-analysis of randomized controlled clinical trials.* JAMA, 1997. **277**(20): 1624.

222. Whelton, P.K., *et al.*, *The effect of potassium supplementation in persons with a high-normal blood pressure: Results from phase I of the Trials of Hypertension Prevention (TOHP).* Annals of Epidemiology, 1995. **5**(2): 85.

223. Swisher, H.E., *Avocado oil: from food use to skin care.* J Amer Oil Chemists' Soc., 1988. **65**: 1704-1706.

224. Tang, R., *et al.*, *Physical activity, water intake and risk of colorectal cancer in Taiwan: a hospital-based case-control study.* International Journal of Cancer, 1999. **82**(4): 484.

225. Michaud, D.S., *et al.*, *Fluid intake and the risk of bladder cancer in men.* New England Journal of Medicine, 1999. **340**(18): 1390.

226. Beyer-Sehlmeyer, G., *Butyrate is only one of several growth inhibitors produced during gut flora-mediated fermentation of dietary fibre sources.* British Journal of Nutrition, 2003. **90**(06): 1057.

227. Ludwig, D.S., *Dietary fiber, weight gain, and cardiovascular disease risk factors in young adults.* JAMA, 1999. **282**(16): 1539.

228. Willett, W.C., *The dietary pyramid: does the foundation need repair?* American Journal of Clinical Nutrition, 1998. **68**: 218.

229. Pentimone, F. and Del Corso, L., *Why regular physical activity favors longevity.* Minerva Medica, 1998. **89**(6): 197-201.

230. Lexell, J., *Human aging, muscle mass, and fiber type composition.* Journals of Gerontology; Series A; Biological Sciences and Medical Sciences, 1995. **50 Spec No**: 11-16.

231. Shimegi, S., *et al.*, *Physical exercise increases bone mineral density in postmenopausal women.* Endocrine Journal, 1994. **41**(1): 49-56.

232. Chandrashekhar, Y. and I. Anand, *Exercise as a coronary protective factor.* American Heart Journal, 1991. **122**(6): 1723.

233. Morris, C.K. and V.F. Froelicher, *Cardiovascular benefits of physical activity.* Herz, 1991. **16**(4): 222-236.

234. Blair, S.N., *et al.*, *Changes in physical fitness and all-cause mortality: a prospective study of healthy and unhealthy men.* JAMA, 1995. **273**(14): 1093.

235. Pate, R.R., *et al.*, *Physical activity and public health: a recommendation from the Centers for Disease Control and Prevention and the American College of Sports Medicine.* JAMA, 1995. **273**(5): 402.

236. Halbert, J., *et al.*, *The effectiveness of exercise training in lowering blood pressure: a meta-analysis of randomised controlled trials of 4 weeks or longer.* J Hum Hypertens, 1997. **11**(10): 641-9.

237. Haskell, W.L., *The influence of exercise on the concentrations of triglyceride and cholesterol in human plasma.* Exercise and Sport Sciences Reviews, 1984. **12**(1): 205.

238. Kantor, M.A., *et al.*, *Exercise acutely increases high density lipoprotein-cholesterol and lipoprotein lipase activity in trained and untrained men.* Metabolism, Clinical and Experimental, 1987. **36**(2): 188.

239. Lokey, E. and Tran, Z., *Effects of exercise training on serum lipid and lipoprotein concentrations in women: a meta-analysis.* Int J Sports Med, 1989. **10**(6): 424-9.

240. Watson, K., Peters, H.A. and Matson, G., *Atherosclerosis in type 2 diabetes mellitus: the role of insulin resistance.* Cardiovasc Pharmacol Ther, 2003. **8**(4): 253-60.

241. Agnarsson, U., *et al.*, *Effects of leisure-time physical activity and ventilatory function on risk for stroke in men: the Reykjavik Study.* Annals of Internal Medicine, 1999. **130**(12): 987.

242. Sacco, R.L., *et al.*, *Leisure-time physical activity and ischemic stroke risk: the Northern Manhattan Stroke Study.* Stroke, 1998. **29**(2): 380.

243. Evenson, K.R., *et al.*, *Physical activity and ischemic stroke risk: the Atherosclerosis Risk in Communities Study.* Stroke, 1999. **30**(7): 1333.

244. Lindsted, K.D., Tonstad, S. and Kuzma, J.W., *Self-report of physical activity and patterns of mortality in Seventh-Day Adventist men.* Journal of Clinical Epidemiology, 1991. **44**(4-5): 355.

245. Manson, J.E., *et al.*, *A prospective study of walking as compared with vigorous exercise in the prevention of coronary heart disease in women.* New England Journal of Medicine, 1999. **341**(9): 650.

246. Henriksen, E., *Invited review: Effects of acute exercise and exercise training on insulin resistance.* Journal of Applied Physiology, 2002. **93**(2): 788-796.

247. Hjeltnes, N., *et al.*, *Exercise-induced overexpression of key regulatory proteins involved in glucose uptake and metabolism in tetraplegic persons: molecular mechanism for improved glucose homeostasis.* FASEB Journal, 1998. **12**(15): 1701.

248. Yki-Järvinen, H., *Kinetics of glucose disposal in whole body and across the forearm in man.* Journal of Clinical Investigation, 1987. **79**(6): 1713.

249. Bak, J.F. and Pedersen, O., *Exercise-enhanced activation of glycogen synthase in human skeletal muscle.* American Journal of Physiology: Endocrinology and Metabolism, 1990. **258**(6): E957.

250. Colditz, G., Cannuscio, C. and Frazier, A., *Physical activity and reduced risk of colon cancer: implications for prevention.* CCC. Cancer Causes & Control, 1997. **8**(4): 649.

251. McTiernan, A., et al., *Physical activity and cancer etiology: associations and mechanisms.* CCC. Cancer Causes & Control, 1998. **9**(5): 487.

252. Friedenreich, C.M., et al., *Epidemiologic issues related to the association between physical activity and breast cancer.* Cancer, 1998. **83**(S3): 600.

253. Courneya, K. and Friedenreich, C., *Physical exercise and quality of life following cancer diagnosis: a literature review.* Annuals of Behavioral Medicine, 1999. **21**(2): 171-179.

254. Dimeo, F.C., et al., *Effects of physical activity on the fatigue and psychologic status of cancer patients during chemotherapy.* Cancer, 1999. **85**(10): 2273.

255. Courneya, K., Mackey, J. and Jones, L., *Coping with cancer.* The Physician and Sports Medicine 2000. **28**: 49-73.

256. Derman, W.E., Coleman, K.L. and Noakes, T.D., *Effects of exercise training in patients with cancer who have undergone chemotherapy.* Medicine and Science in Sports and Exercise, 1999. **31**(5): S368.

257. Mock, V., et al., *Establishing mechanisms to conduct multi-institutional research - fatigue in patients with cancer: an exercise intervention.* Oncology of Nursing Forum 1998. **25**(8): 1391-1397.

258. Glanz, K., *Psychosocial impact of breast cancer: a critical review.* Ann Behav Med, 1992. **14**: 202-212.

259. Ferrell, B.R., *The impact of pain on quality of life. A decade of research*. Nursing Clinics of North America, 1995. **30**(4): 609-624.

260. Morrow, G. and Dobkin, P., *Anticipatory nausea and vomiting in cancer patients undergoing chemotherapy treatment: Prevalence, etiology, and behavioral interventions*. Clinical Psychology Review, 1988. **8**(5): 517.

261. Pelletier, C., Lapointe, L. and LeBlanc, P. *Effects of lung resection on pulmonary function and exercise capacity*. Thorax, 1990. **45**(7): 497.

262. Smith, S.L., *Physical exercise as an oncology nursing intervention to enhance quality of life*. Oncology Nursing Forum, 1996. **23**(5): 771-778.

263. Berkowitz, K.J., *The challenge of exercise: practical advice for implementation into clinical practice*. Nurse Practitioner Forum, 1998. **9**(2): 53-57.

264. Gustafson, N., *Exercising when you're overweight*. Diabetes Self Manage, 1998. **15**(6): 97-8, 100,102.

265. Boule, N., *et al.*, *Effects of exercise on glycemic control and body mass in type 2 diabetes mellitus: a meta-analysis of controlled clinical trials*. JAMA, 2001. **286**(10): 1218.

266. Vestergaard, H., *et al.*, *Glycogen synthase and phosphofructokinase protein and mRNA levels in skeletal muscle from insulin-resistant patients with non-insulin-dependent diabetes mellitus*. Journal of Clinical Investigation, 1993. **91**(6): 2342.

267. Knowler, W., *et al.*, *Reduction in the incidence of type 2 diabetes with lifestyle intervention or metformin*. New England Journal of Medicine, 2002. **346**(6): 393.

268. Despres, J.P., *Visceral obesity, insulin resistance, and dyslipidemia: contribution of endurance exercise training to the*

267

treatment of the plurimetabolic syndrome. Exercise and Sport Sciences Reviews, 1997. **25**: 271.

269. Després, J.P., *Low-intensity endurance exercise training, plasma lipoproteins and the risk of coronary heart disease.* Journal of Internal Medicine, 1994. **236**(1): 7.

270. Mokdad, A.H., *The continuing epidemics of obesity and diabetes in the United States.* JAMA, 2001. **286**(10): 1195.

271. Braunstein, J., *Curtailing a rampant epidemic.* Diabetes Forecast, 2000. **53**(12): 31-33.

272. Segerstrom, S. and Miller, G.E., *Psychological stress and the immune system: A meta analytical study of 30 years of Enquiry.* Psychol Bull, 2004. **130**(4): 601 – 630.

273. Wallace, R. and Wallace, D.N., eds. Structured Psychosocial Stress and the US Obesity Epidemic. 5th ed., 2003, Cornell University Library.

274. Hartvig, K., The Healthy Diet Calorie Counter. 2004.

275. Eriksson, S.F. and Pickova, J., *Fatty acids and tocopherol levels in m. longissimus dorsi of beef cattle in Sweden – a comparison between seasonal diets.* Meat Science, 2007. **76**(4): 746.

276. Clarke, S.D. and Jump, D.B., *Dietary polyunsaturated fatty acid regulation of gene transcription.* Annual Review of Nutrition, 1994. **14**(1): 83.

277. Simopoulos, A.P., *Evolutionary aspects of diet, the omega-6/omega-3 ratio and genetic variation: nutritional implications for chronic diseases.* Biomedicine & Pharmacotherapy, 2006. **60** 502–507.

278. Norris, J.M., et al., *Omega-3 polyunsaturated fatty acid intake and islet autoimmunity in children at increased risk for type 1 diabetes.* JAMA, 2007. **298**(12): 1420.

268

279. Palomba, L., *Inhibition of nitric-oxide synthase-I (NOS-I)-dependent nitric oxide production by lipopolysaccharide plus interferon-γ is mediated by arachidonic acid.* Journal of Biological Chemistry, 2004. **279**(29): 29895.

280. Savva, S.C., et al., *Association of adipose tissue arachidonic acid content with BMI and overweight status in children from Cyprus and Crete.* British Journal of Nutrition, 2004. **91**(04): 643.

281. Korotkova, M., et al., *Gender-related long-term effects in adult rats by perinatal dietary ratio of n-6/n-3 fatty acids.* Regulatory, Integrative, and Comparative Physiology, 2005. **288**(3): R575.

282. Barker, D.J.P., *The origins of the developmental origins theory.* Journal of Internal Medicine, 2007. **261**(5): 412.

Abbreviations and Glossary

Abdominal obesity: the accumulation of fatty tissue around the major organs. It can be considered as an endocrine organ or gland as it secretes hormones and inflammatory proteins into the blood supply. It is a major risk factor for diabetes Type 2 and heart disease.

Acetate: A 2-carbon organic acid formed from the oxidation of ethyl alcohol in vinegar production.

Adipose tissue: fatty body tissue that accumulates the energy-rich triglycerides or fat as energy storage material.

ALA: the essential 18-carbon fatty acid α-linolenic acid. Precursor of the long-chain omega-3 fats which are essential for infant brain and vision development, and cognitive function in the elderly.

Amino acids: Organic acids containing nitrogen that form the building blocks for all proteins.

Amylopectin: highly branched starch molecules which are digested rapidly and can give rise to sudden surges in blood glucose levels.

Amylose: the linear unbranched form of starch which is digested slowly to yield blood glucose.

Aneurism: a sac formed by the abnormal dilation of a weakened blood vessel wall.

AO: antioxidant substances, either natural or synthetic, which can reduce oxidative stress and free radical mediated damage of DNA, protein and membrane lipids.

Apo(a): apoprotein(a) is the sticky protein contained in the lipoprotein(a) transport vesicle that adheres to artery walls and is a risk factor for cardiovascular disease.

Arachidonic acid: the 20-carbon omega-6 fatty acid, formed from linoleic acid and found in animal tissues, which is the parent compound for the proinflammatory series 2 prostaglandins.

Arrhythmia: any variation from the normal rhythm of the heartbeat.

270

Atheroma: an unstable fatty deposit within or on the inner lining of the artery, which can be dislodged to obstruct the blood flow.

Atherosclerosis: a degenerative disease of the inner lining of the artery walls.

ATP: adenosine triphosphate. A high energy compound found in plant and animal mitochondria and all living cells. It is the major source of energy for most cellular reactions.

β-Carotene: a polyunsaturated, orange plant pigment hydrocarbon. It has antioxidant and anticancer properties and acts as a valuable precursor for vitamin A.

Bile acids: natural detergents made from cholesterol in the liver and stored in the gall bladder. They are secreted into the duodenum following a fatty meal where they serve to emulsify the dietary fat prior to its digestion by the pancreatic lipase enzymes in the small intestine.

Butyric acid: a 4-carbon short chain fatty acid found in butter. It is rapidly absorbed and digested without the need for bile acid secretion, and is oxidised for energy rather than being stored in adipose tissue.

Caproic acid: a 6-carbon short chain fatty acid found in tropical oils.

Caprylic acid: an 8-carbon medium chain fatty acid with useful anti-fungal and antibacterial properties. Also found in tropical oils.

Catalase: a protective enzyme which reduces oxidative stress by converting hydrogen peroxide to oxygen and water.

CHD: coronary heart disease. Any heart disorder caused by disease of the coronary arteries.

CVD: cardiovascular disease. A collective term for diseases of the heart and general circulation, including ischaemic heart disease, atherosclerosis and peripheral artery disease.

Cholesterol: a complex waxy sterol with crucial functions in animal cells where it stabilises cell membranes, and acts as a substrate for the synthesis of the steroid hormones and bile acids. In the absence of dietary cholesterol it is readily synthesised in the liver.

Chylomicrons: lipoprotein particles formed in the intestinal cells following a fatty meal. They transport fat and cholesterol via the lymphatic system into the

271

blood stream to be taken up by the adipose tissue and muscle. Digestion in these tissues removes the fatty acids to yield cholesterol-rich remnant particles which are removed and processed in the liver.

Cis-isomer: forms when hydrogen atoms are removed from the same side of a carbon–carbon bond. If this occurs in a long-chain saturated fatty acid, it will introduce a kink into the previously straight chain.

Complex carbohydrates: digestible sugar polymers such as starch and glycogen and indigestible fibres containing cellulose, pectin and hemicelluloses.

DNA: deoxyribonucleic acid. The nucleotide polymer that carries the genetic code for all living things with the exception of the RNA viruses.

DHA: docosahexaenoic acid, a 22-carbon omega-3 fatty acid found in high concentrations in cold water oily fish. It is crucial for infant brain and vision development and may protect brain function in the elderly. It can be synthesised in human cells from the parent short chain omega-3 fatty acid ALA from plant sources.

EPA: eicosapentaenoic acid, a 20-carbon omega-3 fatty acid commonly found in cold water oily fish and marine mammals. EPA is converted to the series 3 prostaglandins which inhibit the inflammatory actions of the series 2 prostaglandins.

EFSA: European Food Standards Agency. A transnational body advised by the food industry to provide recommendations on the composition of processed foods.

Endothelium: the layer of cells surrounding the arterial lumen.

Ester: compounds formed by the reactions of alcohols with acids to eliminate water.

FAO: Food and Agriculture Organization of the United Nations.

FDA: Food and Drug Administration, USA. The government agency controlling the safety of foods and drugs.

Familial hypercholesteraemia: a genetic condition characterised by extremely high concentrations of cholesterol in the blood.

Free radical: extremely reactive atoms or molecules with unpaired electrons.

272

GLA: γ-linolenic acid, an 18-carbon omega-3 fatty acid made from the essential fatty acid linoleate. Found in borage and evening primrose oil and used in the treatment of premenstrual syndrome and arthritis.

Glucagon: this starvation hormone is produced in the pancreas in the absence of dietary carbohydrate. It inhibits fatty acid synthesis, stimulates fat breakdown and stabilises the blood glucose concentration by stimulating glycogen breakdown in the liver.

Glycerol: a 3-carbon alcohol formed from glucose. One glycerol molecule is attached to three fatty acid molecules in a triglyceride (fat) molecule.

Glycogen: a highly branched starch polymer found in animal liver and muscle

g: gram. One thousandth part of a kilogram. One ounce is approximately 28g.

GSH: reduced glutathione; an important antioxidant and cofactor in the regeneration of vitamin C.

HDL: high density lipoprotein is the 'good' cholesterol that interacts with VLDL and LDL to distribute cholesterol in the blood and transfers the excess to the liver for further metabolism or excretion into the bile.

Hydrogenation: the chemical process of catalytically hydrogenating unsaturated triglyceride oils to form spreadable or hard fats. Partial hydrogenation yields toxic industrial trans fats which are now being phased out of processed foods. The complete process yields non-toxic saturated fats.

Hyperlipidaemia: abnormally high levels of lipids, especially cholesterol, in the blood.

Hypertension: high blood pressure.

Hypothalamus: a neural control centre at the base of the brain triggered by hunger, thirst and fear.

IDL: intermediate density lipoprotein. These cholesterol-rich particles are formed following the processing of VLDL in the peripheral tissues and are structurally similar to chylomicron remnant particles. They are either absorbed by the liver or loaded with cholesterol esters from HDL in the circulation to form LDL particles.

Insulin: a protein hormone secreted in the pancreas by the Islets of Langerhans. It lowers excessive blood sugar levels by increasing glucose uptake into muscle and adipose tissue where it stimulates the conversion of glucose to glycogen and fat.

Intima: the space between the endothelium and the smooth muscle wall of an artery or vein, where free radical damage can initiate plaque formation and heart disease.

ITF: industrial trans fat. Formed by partial hydrogenation of polyunsaturated vegetable oils. ITFs are toxic but the biological trans fats in dairy products are either harmless or beneficial in the human diet.

IU: international unit. Agreed unit of measurement for vitamins A, D and E.

Ketones: small water-soluble molecules produced from fat in the liver during carbohydrate deprivation. They are transported to the brain and peripheral tissues where they serve as an alternative energy source to glucose. Examples are β-hydroxybutyrate and acetoacetate.

LA: linoleate is the essential 18-carbon omega-6 fatty acid precursor of the proinflammatory series-2 prostaglandins produced in response to infections. Overconsumption leads to the development of inflammatory conditions such as arthritis and heart disease.

LDL: low density lipoprotein. Cholesterol ester-rich vesicles which deliver fatty acids and cholesterol to growing cells. A rich supply is crucial for infant growth and development. The reference to LDL as 'bad' cholesterol is misleading.

Lipase: an enzyme that specifically breaks down triglycerides to release free fatty acids.

Macrophages: large white phagocytic blood cells occurring also in lymph and body tissues where they can engulf invading microorganisms. They can also take up oxidised LDL to form foam cells which become deposited in arterial plaques.

MCFAs: medium chain fatty acids containing 6–12 carbon atoms. Dietary fats containing these fatty acids are well absorbed and digested for energy and not deposited in body fat.

mM: a millimole is the molecular weight of a substance measured in milligrams. Blood cholesterol is now measured in millimoles per litre or mM/L instead of milligrams per 100 millilitres or mg/dL.

Mitochondria: the small sub-cellular particles that consume oxygen and carry out aerobic respiration in the cells of all higher organisms.

mg: a milligram is one thousandth part of a gram. A convenient unit of measurement for small amounts of material.

NAD: nicotinamide adenine dinucleotide is an essential cofactor involved in the release of energy during the oxidation of sugars and fatty acids in the process of respiration.

NADP: nicotinamide adenine dinucleotide phosphate is the cofactor which traps the energy from respiration and uses it to drive biosynthetic reactions in the cell such as the synthesis of long chain fatty acids.

Necrosis: Cell death and lysis, caused by toxins, which liberates degradative enzymes that can kill surrounding cells.

NO·: nitric oxide. A free radical also referred to as a reactive nitrogen species. It is produced by enzymes in the body where it plays an important role in vasodilation. It is also found as a toxic constituent in smoke and industrial waste gases.

NOS: nitric oxide synthase. The enzyme that produces nitric oxide from the amino acid arginine.

Omega: Greek symbol ω. Used in fatty acid classification to denote the position of a terminal methyl group.

Omega-6 (ω-6): the PUFA family with double bonds starting six carbon atoms from the terminal methyl group. The parent fatty acid linoleate is essential for immune health, but overconsumption can lead to inflammation, obesity and heart disease.

Omega-3 (ω-3): the related PUFAs found in the fat of cold water oily fish and marine mammals. They are precursors for the series-3 prostaglandins which exert an anti-inflammatory effect by inhibiting production of the inflammatory series-2 prostaglandins from the omega-6 PUFAs.

Oxo-LDL: the oxidised derivative of LDL formed during oxidative stress. It binds to a specific receptor on the macrophage. Excessive uptake of oxo-LDL by macrophages leads to the formation of foam cells, which are major risk factors in heart disease.

275

Pituitary gland: the very small but major endocrine gland attached to the base of the brain. Often referred to as the 'director of the endocrine orchestra' as it secretes hormones which control the development of the sex glands, skeletal growth and the functioning of other endocrine glands.

Placebo: an inactive substance or other sham form of therapy administered to a control group of patients to compare the effects with those patients on the real drug or treatment.

PL: phospholipid, the combination of glycerol, two molecules of fatty acid and one phosphate group. Other groups may be attached to the phosphate. The basic structural components of cell membranes and lipoprotein vesicles.

Plaque: a thickening of the artery wall usually initiated by the oxidative free radical damage of LDL cholesterol. Oxo-LDL in the arterial intima stimulates the growth of the surrounding vascular smooth muscle cells to reduce the vessel diameter. Macrophages also bind and engulf oxo-LDL to form foam cells which cluster and adhere to the muscle wall. A proteinaceous skin then forms over the top to yield a stable plaque. If the underlying foam cells burst to liberate lytic enzymes, the plaque may become unstable and rupture to stimulate thrombus formation and blood vessel blockage.

PG: prostaglandin. Partially oxidised intermediates from ω-3 and ω-6 PUFAs with hormone-like functions,which regulate cellular activity.

PPL: postprandial lipaemia. A genetic condition leading to the sluggish clearance of lipids from blood plasma following a fatty meal. An important risk factor in the development of heart disease.

PUFAs: polyunsaturated fatty acids are long chain fatty acids with more than one double bond in the side chain. Two naturally occurring classes of PUFAs are the omega-3 and omega-6 fatty acids, which are essential in the diet.

RDA: Recommended Daily Allowance. The minimum daily dosage of essential nutrients required by the average healthy person to prevent deficiency symptoms. This is not necessarily the optimum dose and takes no account of factors such as body weight, sex, age, metabolic rate and physical activity.

RNA: ribonucleic acid. Polynucleotide molecules which mediate in the transfer of genetic information from DNA into protein structure. Some small RNA molecules are directly involved in the control of gene expression.

RNS: reactive nitrogen species. Highly reactive free radicals such as NO· and non-radicals like peroxynitrite, HONOO⁻.

ROS: reactive oxygen species. Hydroxyl radical (OH·), superoxide (O_2·) and lipid peroxy radicals. Lipid peroxides and hydrogen peroxide are important non-radical ROS.

SOD: superoxide dismutase is a radical scavenging enzyme that partially detoxifies the radical superoxide by converting it to hydrogen peroxide which is subsequently destroyed by catalase.

TG: triglyceride or triacylglycerol (a more accurate description of the molecule) composed of one molecule of glycerol attached by ester bonds to three molecules of fatty acids. The common name is fat. It forms the main energy storage material in fatty or adipose tissue.

Thrombus: a clot of coagulated blood within a blood vessel that may impede or stop the flow of blood.

Trans-isomer: a double bond between carbon atoms with hydrogen atoms attached on the different sides of the bond, to give the molecule a linear shape.

Transesterification: an industrial process for rearranging the fatty acids within triglycerides to alter the melting properties, and replace the toxic ITFs in spreadable fat.

VLDL: very low density lipoprotein. These large TG-rich lipoprotein vesicles are produced in the liver in the absence of adequate dietary fat. They enter the blood and are transported to the peripheral tissues where their TGs are depleted by lipase activity and fatty acids released to form IDL vesicles. The IDL vesicles are then either re-absorbed by the liver or converted to LDL by transfer of cholesterol esters and fatty acids from HDL vesicles in the blood. They are now considered to be as important as LDL vesicles in the prediction of heart disease progression.

277

INDEX

free radicals 42, 114, 141, 229, 230
French paradox 97, 163
fructose 15, 28, 29, 32, 35-38, 93, 227
fruit 6, 9, 11, 29, 30, 37, 48, 52, 53, 56, 61, 65, 72, 92, 147, 156-159, 162, 214, 222-225, 227, 237, 240

gap junction 238
garlic 162
glucagon 15, 20, 92
glucose 14-17, 19, 22-25, 28-30, 37, 39, 40, 43-47, 52, 54, 56, 60, 78, 87, 89, 92, 123, 138, 153, 161, 171, 189-191, 193, 195, 200-205
glucosinolate 161
glutathione 133
glycaemic index (GI) 30, 52, 54, 55
glycaemic load (GL) 30
glycogen 15, 16, 19, 21, 24, 25, 27, 28, 92, 123, 179, 188, 191, 195, 203
G-proteins 120-124
grapes 163

HDL cholesterol 41, 89, 100, 101, 112-116, 119, 129, 134, 160, 172, 187, 188, 217
heart disease 1, 3, 9, 8, 16, 17, 40-42, 69, 96-100, 114, 186
  and dietary fat 97

and protein 75
and ROS 233
hemp 81, 216
high density lipoprotein *see* HDL
high fat diets 25, 26, 96
high protein diet 63, 64, 69
homocysteine 99, 118, 135, 136, 155
HPA 203
human diet 6
hydrogenation 79, 80, 83, 84, 104, 109, 117
hyperinsulinaemia 19
hypoglycaemia 18, 200
hypothalamic–
  pituitary–adrenal axis 203

immune system 39
industrial trans fats 83-90, 94, 104
insulin 15, 17, 19, 44, 46, 68, 87, 101
insulin dependent diabetes
  mellitus 199
insulin resistance 19, 36, 37, 41, 188, 196, 198
interesterified fats 90
Inuit 5, 10, 25, 26, 33, 63, 82, 97, 107, 114, 226
iron 71
ITF *see* industrial trans fats

Japanese diet 71, 122
juice 30
juvenile diabetes 70, 194

283

ubiquinone 122
  see also coenzyme Q10
unsaturated fat 79, 80, 87
unsaturated fatty acids 79

vegetables 3, 8, 10, 30, 37, 45,
  48, 53, 56, 57, 61, 65, 66, 72,
  92, 132, 133, 142, 147, 150,
  156, 157, 159, 162-164, 168,
  213, 220, 224, 225, 237, 240
very low density lipoprotein
  see VLDL
visceral fat 204
vitamin A 131
vitamin B1 133
vitamin B2 133
vitamin B3 133
vitamin B5 134
vitamin B6 135
vitamin B12 135, 136, 155
vitamin C 8, 26, 39, 132, 136-
  139, 143, 144, 158, 160, 225,
  236, 237, 239
vitamin D 108, 131, 134, 140,
  141, 152
vitamin E 141, 142, 144, 145,
  146, 224, 236
vitamin K_1 150
vitamin K_2 141, 151, 153
VLDL 38, 111-113

walnut 81
water quality 167
watercress 161

weight control 68, 179, 198
wine 3, 163
World Health Organisation
  (WHO) 5, 31, 32, 47-51, 57,
  106, 210

xylitol 53, 54, 223

zinc 71, 168

About the authors

Rod Bilton is Professor Emeritus in Applied Biochemistry in the School of Pharmacy and Biomolecular Sciences at Liverpool John Moores University. After his PhD in microbial biochemistry at the University of Newcastle upon Tyne in 1965, he took up an NRDC sponsored post-doctoral fellowship on antibiotic production in the Chemistry Department at Manchester University between 1966 and 1967. He then moved to a Cancer Research Fellowship at Syntex Research in Palo Alto, California. He returned to a lecturing post at the newly formed Liverpool Polytechnic in 1969 and started a research group on steroid biotransformation and mutagenicity testing. A sabbatical year in 1981 sponsored by the Royal Society and the SRC enabled him to work on the latest genetic engineering techniques in the ICI Corporate Bioscience Laboratory. Back at Liverpool Polytechnic, Rod set up a free radical research laboratory to investigate the roles of free radicals and dietary antioxidants in the aetiology of colo-rectal cancer. The chairmanship of a working group on Biomarkers and Mechanisms in an EEC Antioxidant Network Fair 97-3223 provided the impetus for writing this book.

Other duties include grant assessment for the World Cancer Fund and the Wellcome Trust, reviewing for the Gut Journal, and a brief tangle with the legal profession as an Expert Witness for the defence in the Diane Modahl case. Hobbies include the testing of dietary and exercise regimes to battle against the ravages of old age.

Larry Booth graduated with a BSc Hons in Applied Biology at LJMU in 1990 and entered the NHS to qualify as an MLSO with training in microbiology and haematology in Broadgreen, the Royal Liverpool and Walton Hospitals between 1990 and 1993. He returned to Higher Education on a SERC-Case PhD Studentship to research mechanisms of bile acid mediated DNA damage in adenocarcinoma cells. His PhD

286

supervisors were Rod Bilton and Professor Sir Ian Gilmore of the Gastroenterology Unit at the Royal Liverpool University Hospital. He then took a postdoctoral fellowship at Harvard University School of Medicine in the Wellman Laboratories of Photomedicine. He studied the role of photosensitisers using laser light to generate localised reactive oxygen species as potential anti-cancer agents.

Family ties brought him back to the UK in 2004. He obtained his PGCE in 2005 and entered secondary teaching at St. Edwards College Liverpool in the same year. He then moved to a lecturing post at Riverside College in 2007. The lure of original research proved too strong so he returned to the USA in January 2011 to continue with his interests in free radicals and cancer, and to take up a research post in the Massey Cancer Centre, Department of Neurosurgery, Virginia Commonwealth University.

Larry is a passionate supporter of Liverpool Football Club and will be keenly following their renaissance from afar.